MANAGING PROSTATE

CW00706914

MANAGING PROSTATE DISEASE

Professor David Kirk DM FRCS

ALTMAN

Published by Altman Publishing, 7 Ash Copse, Bricket Wood, St Albans, Herts, AL2 3YA

First edition 2007

© 2007 David Kirk

The right of David Kirk to be identified as Author of this Work has been asserted by him in accordance with the Copyright, Designs and Patents Act 1988.

Typeset in 10/12 Optima by Phoenix Photosetting, Chatham, Kent
Printed in Great Britain by Chiltern Printers (Slough) Ltd

ISBN 13: 978-1-86036-036-7

All rights reserved. No part of this publication may be reproduced, stored in a retrieval system or transmitted in any form or by any means, electronic, mechanical, photocopying, recording or otherwise, without the prior written permission of the publisher. Applications for permission should be addressed to the publisher at the address printed on this page.

The publisher makes no representation, express or implied, with regard to the accuracy of the information contained in this book and cannot accept any legal responsibility or liability for any errors or omissions that may be made.

A catalogue record for this book is available from the British Library

∞ Printed on acid-free text paper, manufactured in accordance with ANSI/NISO Z39.48-1992 (Permanence of Paper)

CONTENTS

ABBREVIATIONS

ACT	α1-antichymotrypsin
ACTH	adrenocorticotrophic hormone
BNI	bladder neck incision
BOO	bladder outflow obstruction
BPH	benign prostatic hyperplasia
cPSA	complexed PSA
CT	computed tomography
DRE	digital rectal examination
f/tPSA	ratio of free to total PSA
HIFU	high-intensity focused ultrasound
IMRT	intensity-modulated radiotherapy
IPSS	International Prostate Symptom Score
IVU	intravenous urogram
LH	luteinizing hormone
LHRH	luteinizing hormone releasing hormone
LUTS	lower urinary tract symptoms
α2M	α2-macroglobulin
MR	magnetic resonance
NICE	National Institute for Clinical Excellence
NIH	National Institutes of Health
NSAID	non-steroidal anti-inflammatory drug
PAC	prostate assessment clinic
PIN	prostatic intra-epithelial neoplasia
PSA	prostate specific antigen
PSAD	prostate specific acid density
PSAV	prostate specific acid velocity
RPP	retropubic prostatectomy
RU	residual urine
TRUS	transurethral ultrasound
TUIP	transurethral incision of prostate
TURP	transurethral resection of the prostate
UICC	International Union Against Cancer
UTI	urinary tract infection

ABOUT THE AUTHOR

David Kirk recently retired from his appointment as Consultant Urologist at Gartnavel General Hospital, Glasgow. He was also an Honorary Professor, University of Glasgow, and Lead Urologist, North Glasgow University Hospitals Trust. His principal clinical and research interests were in management and investigation of urological cancer, especially of prostatic carcinoma and tumours of the testis. As the founding Chairman of the Prostate Forum, he was among the first to be involved in the development of shared care protocols in managing prostatic disease. Among his publications is 'Understanding Prostate Disorders', a popular information booklet for patients.

ABOUT THIS BOOK

Prostate disorders have become recognized as an important health issue in the care of middle-aged and elderly men. Improved methods of diagnosing prostate cancer have dramatically increased the incidence of recognized disease, yet have created a number of dilemmas in its management. As medical treatment has become available for benign prostatic enlargement, so has the perspective of this condition altered. These changes have had an inevitable impact on the primary care team. There is increasing scope for diagnosis and management of prostate disorders within the community, and such a shift is encouraged by current policies in health-care delivery. The main function of this book is to improve the confidence of the primary care team, general practitioners and practice nurses, in dealing with men with prostate disease. The author hopes that it will also be useful for specialist nurses, working in urology departments, who play an increasing role in the management of men with prostate disorders. It may also provide a useful introduction to the subject for doctors considering or embarking on a career in urology.

ACKNOWLEDGEMENTS

I should like to thank several colleagues for their assistance: Mr David Hendry and Professor Richard Simpson, for their helpful comments on the text, and my nursing colleagues, Mrs Cathy McClean and Ms Bria McAllister. Any errors and omissions are solely my responsibility.

1 INTRODUCTION

Over the quarter of a century during which the author has practised urology, there has been a sea change in the management of prostate disease. Before then, the only active intervention (other than catheterization) for benign prostatic enlargement was surgery. Even this was a hit and miss affair without the refinements of urodynamics – indeed, many men went to surgery without even a simple urine flow measurement. Prostate cancer was usually diagnosed at an advanced stage when all that could be offered was hormonal therapy or, occasionally, palliative radiotherapy. It is quite possible that no one in the UK underwent a radical prostatectomy in the 1970s. Public perception of prostate disease has changed. Its symptoms in the past were largely a cause of humour – witness Private Godfrey in the sitcom 'Dad's Army' with his frequent requests to be able to 'have a run out'. Fear of surgery, embarrassment and a feeling that the problem was simply a matter of getting old led to many men putting up with their symptoms.

Then, in the 1990s, the prostate was discovered by the media. Articles on prostate disease now feature regularly in newspapers and magazines; inevitably these focus on cancer, always the more newsworthy condition. Men with minor symptoms, worried about cancer, queue up to seek reassurance. Others (or, often, their wives) now realize treatment is possible for their symptoms. This heightened public awareness has occurred when there has been a steady increase in the elderly population. This, and improved diagnostic methods, have increased the incidence of prostate cancer. Preventive medicine is encouraging regular health checks, whether within the NHS primary care service, or commercially. How important is looking for prostate disease in these checks? Finally, there is now effective medical treatment for symptoms due to benign prostatic enlargement. Management no longer always requires the skills of a surgeon, creating opportunities for managing men in primary care. All this has happened at a time when hospital services are under increasing pressure and when health policy is directed to moving care into the community, where this is safe and cost-effective.

The increasing numbers of men consulting about 'prostate problems' will affect practice nurses as much as general practitioners. The complexity and choice in management of, for example, early prostate cancer, about which many men will seek advice from their general practitioner, in itself creates an increasing burden for the primary care team. However, there are also now opportunities for the committed health-care team to take on the diagnosis and management of the many men with lower urinary symptoms who do not require the specialist intervention of the urologist, and to prioritize the referral of those who do. Even in the management of prostate cancer, sharing care between the specialist urologist or oncologist and the primary care team can only benefit the patient.

The aim of the author in writing this book has not been to provide a comprehensive compendium on prostate disease, but to highlight those issues that will help with the inevitable consultations by men with lower urinary symptoms and with concerns about prostate cancer, and to facilitate management in primary care when this is appropriate. The decisions to be made following the introduction of 'Patient Choice' into the NHS in England will also require the patient to be informed of the rationale behind secondary care management.

A note on the text

Older, but perhaps familiar terms, which inappropriately imply an aetiology that may not be the cause, have been discarded. For example, 'lower urinary tract symptoms (LUTS)' has replaced 'prostatism' or 'prostatic symptoms'; 'pelvic pain syndrome' is used instead of 'prostatitis'. These current terms will be used in this book.

Logically, benign and malignant disease of the prostate should be considered separately, and to an extent this has been done. However, the two are intrinsically linked, not least in the minds of many of our patients. Distinguishing between the two is an essential part of the initial assessment of the patient, even in those with symptoms most likely to be due to benign disease. Some sections will clearly be relevant to both; if, as a result, there has been some repetition in other parts of the book, this has been done in the interests of clarity.

2 SETTING THE SCENE

'I am having to get up to pass urine three times each night, doctor. Is this serious?'

Management of most illnesses starts in the primary care consulting room. Perhaps the majority of men over 60 will, on questioning, have at least mild lower urinary symptoms. These may themselves be the reason for consultation, or come to light incidentally, either 'while I'm here, doctor' or as a result of direct enquiry from the doctor or nurse. Although many men with mild symptoms do not require treatment, in the past men did often suppress troublesome symptoms as one of the inevitable consequences of old age. Indeed, it is still often the patient's wife who initiates the consultation. Once the symptoms come to light, questions arise, questions which may concern the doctor as much as his patient

'Can you do anything to make me better?'
'What is the cause of the symptoms?' – or, perhaps, more commonly,
'Do I have cancer, doctor?'
'Will the trouble make me ill in the future?'

The prostate may intrude into practice in other ways. Acute retention of urine is among the commoner surgical emergencies, and chronic retention is an uncommon, but, because it is reversible, important cause of renal failure. While prostate cancer may present with, or come to light during investigation of, lower urinary symptoms, it may also present with bone pain or other manifestations of metastases. Requests for a prostate specific antigen (PSA) test are an increasing feature of both primary care and urological practice. Should men be offered a PSA test as part of a routine 'health check-up'?

This is a guidebook for the primary care team for the journey on which they will embark with the patient following this initial consultation. As with all journeys, a map is needed. The next few chapters provide the background material on which the management of prostatic disease is based. The journey will then be described, with most detail in those areas where the patient can be managed in primary care. For some, much of the journey will take place in secondary care. Here, the emphasis is different, concentrating on important material to enable the inevitable questions and concerns of patients to be answered, to alert the primary care team to the indications for intervention and referral, and to encourage the shared care approach to prostate disease that has come to benefit patients with so many other conditions.

The text is in two parts. 'Management points' can be looked on as the itinerary for the journey, presenting in a didactic form basic information for everyday use. The fuller text is the guidebook, providing detailed explanation and background material. This may be read at leisure, but should not require repeated re-reference.

3 THE PROSTATE – WHAT IS IT AND WHAT DOES IT DO?

to is
·vini
·h gn

Management points

- The prostate lies deep in the pelvis. Relationships important to the surgeon – the bladder sphincters, nerves to the penis, blood vessels and the rectum – are important for understanding the potential complications of treatment.
- The anatomy of the prostate is best understood in terms of its zones, rather than the traditional 'lobes', which are a surgeon's description of the enlarged prostate. These zones have different pathological significance. Benign prostatic hyperplasia (BPH) invariably affects, and is confined to, the transitional zone. Eighty per cent of carcinomas arise in the peripheral zone.
- Internal and external sphincters, above and below the prostate, control the bladder outflow. The internal sphincter at the bladder neck also controls normal ejaculation.
- The prominent stroma of the prostate contains a substantial amount of smooth muscle, important in the aetiology and treatment of bladder outflow obstruction (BOO).
- The prostate produces much of the seminal fluid, which is the source of prostate specific antigen (PSA), a substance unique to the prostate.
- The secretions of the prostate are acidic; this has some therapeutic significance in management of infections – see Chapter 19.

Anatomy of the prostate

Many men, even if they have heard of the prostate, have little idea of where it is or what it does.

Position and relationships

The prostate lies immediately below the bladder (Figure 3.1). The muscle surrounding the bladder neck (internal sphincter) is closely applied almost to the point of merger with the prostate. In addition to its function in controlling the urine within the bladder, the internal bladder sphincter is essential for normal ejaculation, closing to prevent both reflux of semen into the bladder, and also leakage of urine through the relaxed external sphincter. Related to this function is its very rich adrenergic innervation, which is not present in the female bladder neck. Surrounding the urethra in the distal prostate and below is a condensation of muscle which merges with the pelvic floor. Integrity of this 'external sphincter' can maintain continence even if the internal sphincter is destroyed.

The nerves controlling erection lie on either side of the prostate, and are at risk during prostatic surgery. Also of importance to the surgeon is the dorsal vein of the penis which lies anterior to the apex of the gland and can be a source of severe intra-operative bleeding. Posteriorly, the rectum is separated by Denonvillier's fascia.

Anyone who has managed a man with clot retention after prostatic surgery will be aware of the rich blood supply of the gland, which comes

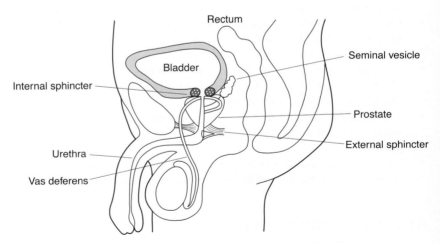

Figure 3.1 Anatomy of the prostate – cross-section of pelvis showing its position and relationships.

from the vesical arteries. Appreciation of the relationship of the prostatic arteries to the penile nerves is critical in maintaining erectile function following surgery. Venous drainage into the paravertebral veins may in part explain the distribution of distant metastases from prostate cancer. Lymphatic drainage is into the iliac and obturator groups of nodes.

The prostatic ducts, vas deferens and the seminal vesicles open into the urethra on either side of a prominence on its posterior wall, the verumontanum. This structure is, for the urologist, an important landmark identifying the upper end of the external sphincter complex.

The prostate, deep in the pelvis, is relatively inaccessible to the surgeon. Abdominal access is normally achieved through the retropubic space, or via the bladder ('suprapubic' or 'transvesical'). The prostate can also be exposed through the perineum, and a rarely used posterior approach, pushing aside the rectum, is described. The majority of operations for benign disease are done endoscopically via the urethra, and laparoscopic procedures are rapidly finding a role, particularly in managing cancer.

Zones of the prostate

Urologists traditionally have described lateral and middle 'lobes' of the prostate; these refer to the appearance of the pathologically enlarged gland (Figure 3.2) and in the normal gland have no anatomical or physiological significance. In some animal species, there are two pairs of glands

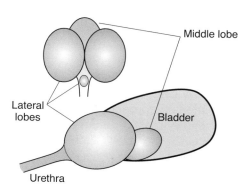

Figure 3.2 Anatomy of the prostate – lobes of the enlarged gland.

opening into the posterior urethra. In the human these have merged into a single glandular structure which surrounds the urethra and the neck of the bladder. Anatomically this origin from two glands can still be identified, and as a result the prostate can be divided into a number of zones (Figure 3.3). Presumably they serve different functions; more importantly, they are the sites of different diseases. In particular, the transitional zone is the site of benign hyperplasia to which it is confined, while 80% of cancers develop in the peripheral zone.

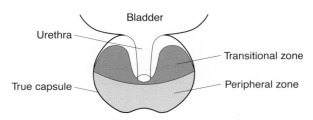

Figure 3.3   Anatomy of the prostate – zones.

Structure of the prostate

In addition to its glandular epithelium, the prostate has a prominent stroma, notable for its content of smooth muscle. Interaction at the molecular biological level between glands and stroma are recognized as important in the pathophysiology of prostatic diseases.

Function of the prostate

The prostate gland produces a substantial part of the seminal fluid, essential for the regulation of reproduction. As a reflection of its specialized function, its secretions contain a number of unique substances. In managing prostate disease, the most significant of these is 'prostate specific antigen (PSA)', the subject of a later section of this book. This has a clearly defined physiological role. As a protease enzyme it breaks down the seminal coagulum which forms after ejaculation, allowing the release of sperms into the cervix. For practical purposes, PSA is only produced

8

by the prostate, hence its specificity in the investigation and management of prostatic disease. Older readers will recall that the marker for prostate cancer which preceded the introduction of PSA was acid phosphatase, and the acidic pH of the prostatic secretions is of significance in relation to antibiotic therapy (see Chapter 19).

4 WHAT CAN GO WRONG?

Enlargement of the prostate is one of the commonest conditions afflicting the male and prostate cancer is among the commonest of malignancies. Inflammatory disease and related conditions (pelvic pain syndrome) occur in young and old and may be more common than is often appreciated.

Benign prostatic hyperplasia

Management points

- Benign prostatic hyperplasia (BPH) starts to develop around age 50 and affects the majority of elderly men.
- Enlargement of the prostate is not in itself significant. A very large prostate may cause few symptoms; a small one may be very troublesome.
- Symptoms from BPH result when it causes bladder outflow obstruction (BOO).
- Lower urinary tract symptoms (LUTS) rather than 'prostatism' is the preferred term for describing these symptoms.
- Voiding (preferred to 'obstructive') symptoms – poor stream, hesitancy, straining and incomplete bladder emptying – are directly attributable to obstruction.
- Storage symptoms (preferred to 'irritative') symptoms – frequency, nocturia, urgency, urge incontinence, sensation of incomplete bladder emptying with an empty bladder – are due to bladder instability (overactive bladder).
- When storage symptoms are secondary to bladder outflow obstruction, these usually resolve after transurethral resection of the prostate (TURP) or other treatment.
- Symptoms from instability (overactive bladder) without obstruction may be aggravated by surgery. Caution is needed in recommending surgery to the man with incontinence, unless due to retention with overflow.

- HAEMATURIA MUST BE INVESTIGATED BY URGENT REFERRAL and not assumed to be due to prostate disease.
- Acute retention is painful; the pain is instantly relieved by catheterization. The volume of urine in the bladder is <900 ml.
- Chronic retention with low pressure may reach 2–3 litres. It may be relatively asymptomatic, or present with LUTS.
- Chronic retention with overflow is an important cause of incontinence in the elderly.
- Acute-on-chronic retention describes painful retention, when urine volume >1000 ml.
- High pressure chronic retention can lead to renal failure.

Other complications

- Urinary infection. May be due to a high residual urine volume, although recurrent infection is often due to inadequately treated prostatitis (see Chapter 19).
- Bladder stones.
- Diverticula – when small, they are of no great clinical significance. Large ones can cause problems, but results from their removal are often disappointing.

Differential diagnosis – other causes of obstruction

- Bladder neck stenosis and urethral stricture are particularly to be suspected when symptoms occur in a younger man.
- Bladder tumour invading bladder neck will usually be associated with haematuria.
- Bladder stones cause intermittent obstruction, often associated with urethral pain.

Differential diagnosis – other urinary disease

- Bladder cancer is to be suspected with sudden onset of storage symptoms, especially if frank or microscopic haematuria is present.
- Renal failure with polyuria.
- Neurological disease (strokes, multiple sclerosis, neuropathies, etc.) affecting the bladder.
- Central disc prolapse or spinal tumours may present with retention of urine.

Differential diagnosis – non-urological disease

- Diseases that cause polyuria – diabetes, early renal failure, diuretic therapy, etc.
- Chronic alcohol and drug abuse may cause bladder dysfunction.
- Abnormal fluid intake.
- 'Ageing' – multiple factors: failing renal function, poor sleep pattern, reduced bladder compliance, behavioural problems associated with dementia.

Pathology of benign prostatic enlargement

Enlargement of the prostate is an event associated with ageing. It usually starts to develop around the age of 50. Its aetiology remains a subject of research, but is probably related to hormonal changes affecting the relative proportions of androgens and oestrogens which occur at that age. Whether a condition ubiquitously related to the ageing process should be called a 'disease' can be questioned, but *benign prostatic hyperplasia* (BPH) is a definite histopathological condition and should not be dismissed simply as 'part of getting old'.

BPH occurs in, and is confined to, the transitional zone of the prostate (see p. 7, 'Zones of the prostate'). As the enlargement increases, it attenuates the overlying peripheral zone. Urologists refer to the stretched peripheral zone as 'the capsule', although the true anatomical capsule of the prostate is a thin, ill-defined structure surrounding the peripheral zone. In traditional open surgery for benign disease, the enlarged portion is extracted by enucleation from within this surgical 'capsule'. It is important to appreciate that even complete removal of the benignly enlarged tissue, although erroneously described as a 'prostatectomy', leaves behind a substantial portion of the prostate, which, critically, is the very part of the gland in which cancer usually develops.

The histopathological changes of BPH can be present without the gland being enlarged. The size of the prostate in itself is relatively unimportant. Considerable enlargement can occur without any ill effects and investigation and treatment simply because the prostate is enlarged is unnecessary. Equally, severe effects can occur with little or no actual increase in size. However, the size of the gland does influence the choices when treatment is needed.

BPH produces its ill effects by blocking the bladder neck and prostatic urethra – *bladder outflow obstruction* (BOO) – which can cause a variety of symptoms. This has two components, mechanical blockage from encroachment of the enlarging tissue into the prostatic urethra and functional obstruction from the activity of the prostatic smooth muscle and bladder neck.

Classification and pathogenesis of lower urinary tract symptoms in the male

The old term 'prostatism' has been replaced by *lower urinary tract symptoms* (LUTS), which does not imply a particular aetiology. Symptoms used to be sub-classified as either *obstructive* or *irritative*. Although these terms are still widely used, *voiding* and *storage* are now to be preferred, and will be used throughout this book.

Voiding symptoms

If due to prostatic disease, the immediate cause of symptoms is obstruction of the urethra. This results in a *deterioration of the urinary stream, hesitancy,* a need to *strain* or to relax the pelvic floor, and awareness of *incomplete emptying* of the bladder. Voiding symptoms are easy to understand on the basis of occlusion of the urethra by an enlarged prostate.

Storage symptoms

These symptoms, *frequency, nocturia* and *urgency,* are more difficult to explain, are less specific and yet may be the greatest cause of distress. Note that a feeling of *incomplete bladder emptying,* when there is not a significant residual urine, can be a storage symptom. It is important to distinguish between true frequency, i.e. frequent passage of small urine volumes, and *polyuria* due to diuresis, where large urine volumes are passed.

Although some men complain of non-specific discomfort passing urine, true, burning, dysuria is not a symptom of uncomplicated BOO, and suggests a urinary infection or prostatitis, or a bladder stone. Finally, haematuria should NEVER be assumed due to prostatic disease until bladder (or renal) cancer has been excluded by appropriate investigation following urgent referral.

Post-micturition dribble

Dribbling urine after voiding is common when the urinary stream is slow and prolonged due to BOO. However, some men experience a troublesome dribble in the absence of other symptoms, often starting in the 40s or 50s, i.e. before the usual age for BOO due to BPH. This is *not* a symptom of obstruction, but probably results from a combination of reduced compliance of the urethra and weakness of the pelvic floor muscles, allowing urine to accumulate in the urethra. It will not be helped by treatment for BPH, certainly not by surgery which can actually cause post-micturition dribbling. 'Milking' the urethra after voiding may help, as may pelvic floor exercises. However, explanation of the benign nature of the symptom, and encouraging patience before 'zipping up', may be all that is necessary.

What happens to the bladder?

The thick-walled, trabeculated bladder with its saccules and diverticula, found in a man with prolonged severe BOO (see Figure 4.1) is the irreversible consequence of prolonged obstruction. When obstruction begins, the bladder is affected, at first functionally, and in different ways. In some cases, it weakens and stretches, ultimately leading to *chronic retention*. In others, the bladder adapts by increasing the voiding pressure, which at first may mask the symptoms but in the long term this can result in high pressure retention leading to renal failure. The commonest outcome, and the usual cause of storage symptoms, is characterized by abnormal waves of increased pressure during bladder filling. This is usually described as *bladder instability*, although the term *overactive bladder* may now be preferred. Unless it is long-standing, instability secondary to obstruction can be reversible, and will improve

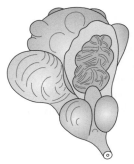

Figure 4.1   Bladder in advanced BOO, showing trabeculation, saccules and diverticula.

15

in the majority of men after relief of obstruction, but *only if obstruction is the cause.*

In the past, all urinary symptoms in elderly men tended to be blamed on 'the prostate' and many inappropriate prostate operations were performed. With the methods of assessment of bladder function now available, we can identify those for whom treatment for obstruction, be it medical or surgical, is appropriate. *Patients must be clear that referral is in the first instance for diagnosis and, to avoid undue expectation, that an operation is not always the appropriate solution.*

Complications of bladder outflow obstruction

Retention of urine

Acute retention, the sudden inability to pass urine, is characterized by pain, relieved almost instantly by catheterization. There will be a relatively low volume of urine (<900 ml) in the bladder. It may be preceded by episodes of severe hesitancy or transient retention. It can be precipitated by surgery (especially lower abdominal, groin or anorectal procedures) or even simply being confined to bed. Over-distension of the bladder, either because of lack of access to a toilet, or the result of a large (especially alcoholic) fluid intake or prescription of diuretics can tip a man into retention, as can constipation.

Chronic retention is painless. If the bladder wall becomes weaker, an increasing amount of urine (*residual*) remains after voiding. When this residual becomes larger than the normal bladder capacity (400–500 ml), it can be defined as chronic retention; the bladder may ultimately reach a volume of several litres. Some patients are completely unaware of this (except perhaps for the need to buy larger trousers!). The distended bladder may only be discovered on examination. More often, the patient presents with urinary frequency or, paradoxically, overflow incontinence – always check for a large bladder in a man who wets himself. Painful retention sometimes supervenes. *Acute-on-chronic retention* should be suspected if more than a litre of urine drains when the patient is catheterized.

High-pressure chronic retention is less common but important as it can be complicated by hydronephrosis and renal failure (Figure 4.2). Because of the high pressure, the patient may be unaware of any voiding symptoms. A fairly specific symptom of high-pressure chronic retention is nocturnal incontinence.

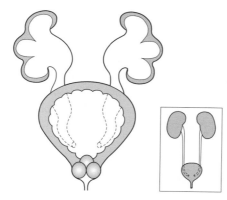

Figure 4.2 Chronic retention with hydronephrosis.

A rare presentation of chronic retention is lower limb oedema due to the distended bladder compressing the pelvic veins – an alarming finding which might incorrectly suggest malignancy (see p. 22 'Symptoms and consequences of prostate cancer').

Urinary infection
When there is a high residual urine, it will be prone to infection. However, many infections in elderly men are due to relapsing prostatitis (Chapter 19), and prostatic surgery is not always the answer.

Incontinence
While urge incontinence from severe instability with proven BOO and overflow incontinence from chronic retention are indications for prostatic surgery, extreme caution is necessary as inappropriate surgery might only make the situation worse.

Bladder stones
As with infection, these tend to be associated with high residual urine, preventing debris and small particles from being cleared from the bladder. Occasionally a renal calculus passed into the bladder spontaneously will be retained and increase in size. More frequently the nidus for the stone is a small calculus released from the prostate itself.

Diverticula

Small saccules and diverticula are common in the elderly man's bladder and may result from obstruction (see Figure 4.1). They are usually of little importance but occasionally a large diverticulum can act as a 'sump' and cause infection or even a calculus. Removal may be indicated in these circumstances although the results can be disappointing. A true diverticulum does not have a muscular wall. If a bladder tumour develops in one, prompt treatment, usually involving diverticulectomy, is essential to prevent early progression.

Differential diagnosis

If the symptoms produced by the prostate are non-specific, what might be alternative causes?

Other causes of obstruction

Bladder neck hypertrophy is a variant of BOO. It can occur in younger men and should be thought of when symptoms are long-standing. A bladder neck stricture or fibrotic stenosis can be a complication of prostatic surgery, including radical prostatectomy done for cancer.

Bladder cancer involving the bladder neck can present with voiding symptoms, usually associated with haematuria.

Bladder stones typically cause intermittent obstruction, classically associated with referred pain from the bladder trigone in the tip of the penis.

Urethral stricture should be suspected in the young man with obstruction (although it can present at any age), especially if there is a history of urethritis, trauma, or urethral instrumention or catheterization, and is also a complication of prostatic surgery.

Other urinary disease

Bladder cancer can present with storage symptoms – a sudden onset of such symptoms, especially when there is occult (chemical or micro-scopic) haematuria, is an indication for cystoscopy to exclude bladder cancer. Frank haematuria is always an indication for investigation. Although a large benign prostate can bleed, it is never safe to assume this to be the case. Haematuria is only a rare presentation of prostate carcinoma.

In the early stages of *renal failure*, the ability to concentrate urine is lost and may result in frequency and, especially, nocturia.

Neurological disease can affect the bladder in a number of ways. Neuropathic bladder instability can occur after strokes, in multiple sclerosis or with neuropathies (alcohol, diabetes, etc.), which can also cause detrusor muscle weakness or incontinence. Retention of urine due to spinal cord or cauda equina compression from disc disease or spinal tumours is a neurosurgical emergency.

Urinary symptoms due to non-urological disease

In an elderly man, urinary frequency is all too readily blamed on 'the prostate'. However, there are many conditions which produce an increased volume of urine output (*polyuria*), with the inevitable consequence of frequency. *Diabetes mellitus* causing frequency is sometimes first picked up in the urology clinic but other conditions can cause polyuria – *diabetes insipidus, early renal failure, diuretic therapy*, etc. *Alcohol abuse* not only has diuretic effects, but also in the long term can affect the bladder through neurological damage. Drug abusers can develop bladder dysfunction. Physiological polyuria due to high fluid intake may not be the sole cause of symptoms, but its correction may be sufficient to avoid more aggressive treatment. The typical syndrome is the recently retired man who starts to drink more tea and coffee, and takes an unaccustomed pint in the local at lunchtime.

As with most systems, urinary function cannot escape the effects of ageing – impaired renal function, disordered sleep pattern, deteriorating bladder compliance, dementia can all combine to cause LUTS in both sexes.

It is also worth noting the potential diagnostic confusion between urinary retention and *anuria* or *oliguria* due to dehydration, ureteric obstruction, acute renal failure, etc.

Adenocarcinoma of the prostate

Management points

- Most tumours occur in the peripheral zone of the prostate, invading beyond the prostate while asymptomatic and causing LUTS only when advanced. Prostate cancer is not eradicated or prevented by transurethral resection of the prostate (TURP), and may not be diagnosed from TURP chips. When early cancer is diagnosed in a man with LUTS, the symptoms are usually due to coincidental BPH.
- Clinical prostate cancer is rare below age 50. Occult cancer is found on post mortem in 30% of men over age 50. Detectable prostate cancer is often asymptomatic and even men presenting with symptomatic disease often die from other causes.
- Locally advanced prostate cancer may present with LUTS, with retention of urine, with ureteric obstruction causing renal failure or in advanced cases, with lower limb oedema due to lymphatic or venous obstruction.
- Lymphatic metastases in the pelvis are difficult to diagnose without biopsy. When extensive, they may cause oedema or ureteric obstruction. Prostate cancer occasionally presents with supraclavicular or other distant lymphadenopathy.
- Distant metastases usually start in the pelvic bones and vertebrae. Early metastases are detectable on bone scan or MR imaging. When visible on x-ray, bone metastases usually are sclerotic. The typical presentation is with back pain, and occasionally with spinal cord compression or pathological fracture. Lung and liver metastases are uncommon and usually occur late in the disease. Brain metastases are extremely rare.

Pathology and epidemiology of prostate cancer

Although the prostate can, rarely, be the site of other primary or secondary tumours, for practical purposes, cancer of the prostate is an adenocarcinoma. Eighty per cent of tumours develop in the peripheral zone. This has a number of important implications.

- A small tumour is likely to be asymptomatic. By the time a peripheral zone tumour has encroached sufficiently into the centre of the gland to obstruct the urethra, it will have reached an advanced and probably incurable stage.

- Thus, a tumour often will invade the capsule and periprostatic tissues while still asymptomatic.
- Although the onset of lower urinary symptoms often initiates the investigations that diagnose cancer, unless the cancer is advanced, these symptoms are usually due to coincidental BPH rather than the tumour itself.
- Transurethral resection of transitional zone BPH may not diagnose a coincidental cancer in the peripheral zone; neither it, nor indeed a traditional open 'prostatectomy', will prevent such a tumour developing later.

Prostatic intra-epithelial neoplasia (PIN), particularly of high grade, is a probable precursor of invasive cancer. Not in itself sufficient to demand treatment, if present on biopsy without invasive malignancy, it would be an indication for further biopsy (see Chapter 13).

Classic post mortem studies have shown that histological foci of adeno-carcinoma can be found in the prostates of 30% of men over 50, and in almost all who survive to 90 (Figure 4.3). These tumours can appear as early as the fourth decade of life. While the natural history of such microscopic tumours is to develop into invasive cancer, this process takes

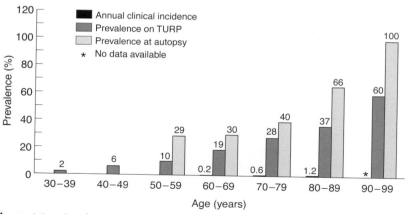

Figure 4.3 Graph showing age incidence of occult CaP, lower urinary symptoms, clinical cancer of the prostate and mortality, by age.

place over many years and will not lead to clinical disease in a majority of men. The prevalence of this occult disease appears to be uniform around the world. The wide geographical variations in the incidence of the clinical disease probably result from factors (environmental, racial, etc.) affecting progression from occult to overt prostate cancer.

In practice, prostate cancer is uncommon under the age of 50, and really should not be considered as a diagnosis in someone under 40. However, there is a genetic predisposition in some men – *familial prostate cancer* – which typically can occur at a younger age. This is suspected when the disease has occurred in a number of first-degree relatives, particularly if their disease occurred at a young age. Having a single relative probably constitutes only a slight increase in risk. Black races, who seem to be at greater risk and in whom the disease may be more aggressive, also are at risk from a younger age.

Symptoms and consequences of prostate cancer

Advanced prostate cancer may cause BOO and present with similar symptoms to BPH, traditionally thought to be of more rapid onset. The author has not found this a useful distinction as men with prostate cancer frequently have pre-existing BPH causing lower urinary symptoms. Additional manifestations of prostate cancer result from local invasion and distant metastases.

Locally advanced disease

In addition to lower urinary symptoms, the advancing cancer can cause venous and lymphatic or ureteric obstruction. Invasion of the rectum is usually a late manifestation, but advanced terminal prostate cancer occasionally causes bowel obstruction. Invasion into the rectal lumen is unusual; a prostato-rectal fistula is more likely when there has been radiotherapy treatment. Occasionally the distinction between a rectal primary and invasion from the prostate is dependent on biopsy findings. In its final stages, a 'frozen pelvis' with encasement of rectum and bladder by tumour can produce an intractable and distressing situation.

Lymphatic metastases

Spread of tumour to regional lymph nodes is normally insidious, although its detection can be important in planning treatment of early disease. Advanced lymphatic metastases can cause lower limb oedema or ureteric obstruction with renal failure. Distant lymphatic metastases (usually in the supraclavicular fossa) at presentation are usually diagnosed after biopsy.

Distant metastases

Predominantly, prostate cancer metastasizes to the bones of the axial skeleton. When visible on radiology the metastases are typically osteoblastic (i.e. sclerotic – Figure 4.4). Differentiation from benign conditions such as Paget's disease can sometimes be difficult. Early metastases not visible on x-ray are detectable on bone scintigraphy or on MR or CT scans. Vertebral metastases can advance to cause spinal cord compression, and despite their sclerotic appearance, pathological fractures occur. In a man suspected of bony metastatic disease, or presenting with unexplained back pain, excluding prostatic cancer is essential, as this is one of the few cancers for which effective treatment is

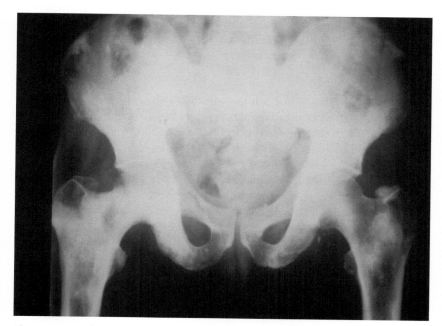

Figure 4.4   Sclerotic metastases from cancer of prostate.

available for disease at this advanced stage. The role of PSA measurement in this context is discussed in the next chapter. In difficult cases a bone biopsy may be needed.

Metastases at other sites – lung or liver – are normally a feature of terminal disease, and are unusual in the absence of associated bony metastases. An infiltrative form of lung metastases can occasionally present with respiratory symptoms. Brain metastases are extremely rare, but neurological symptoms occasionally result from compression or infiltration by a skull metastasis. In the prostate cancer age group, neurological symptoms are much more likely to be due to other disease, e.g. cerebrovascular, degeneration, or metastases from a second tumour.

'Carcinomatosis'

In an old man who is demonstrating generalized debility or weight loss, undisclosed malignancy is obviously an important differential diagnosis. As a readily available diagnostic test, PSA is often measured in this situation. Sadly, the results may be equivocal (see Chapters 5 and 12). Generally speaking, it would be unusual for prostate cancer to present in this way without readily demonstrable bony metastases. An exception to this statement would be debilitation, not due to metastases, but from renal failure resulting from ureteric obstruction by locally advanced disease.

Coincidental prostate cancer

As one of the commonest malignancies, prostate cancer can occur in the presence of other conditions. It is not uncommon for a man with another form of cancer to coincidently have early and irrelevant localized prostate cancer – a conundrum that can cause considerable diagnostic difficulty. Sufficient at this point to emphasize that in these circumstances, finding prostate cancer may not be the end of the story, and should not blind the investigator to other possible causes of the patient's condition.

Prostatitis/pelvic pain syndromes

Management points

- Acute prostatitis presents with severe LUTS and symptoms and signs of systemic infection.
- Milder forms can be confused with simple urinary infection.
- 'Chronic prostatitis' has been abandoned as a descriptive term in favour of 'pelvic pain syndrome' which is described in detail in Chapter 19.

Acute infection of the prostate produces severe lower urinary symptoms, high fever with, on examination, an acutely tender prostate. Rarely, an abscess may develop. Acute infective prostatitis may be associated with epididymo-orchitis (infection spreading via the vas deferens), symptoms of which may mask those from the prostate itself. Chronic but symptomatic infection or inflammation of the prostate causes less clear symptoms; similar ones can occur without evidence of inflammation. The term 'chronic prostatitis' has now been replaced by 'pelvic pain syndrome'. The diagnostic and treatment issues raised by these common but difficult conditions are dealt with in Chapter 19. At this point, it is sufficient to record the importance of considering and adequately treating possible prostatitis in a man with a 'urinary infection'.

5 PROSTATE SPECIFIC ANTIGEN (PSA)

- Prostate specific antigen as a diagnostic test for prostate cancer has poor specificity.
- A 'normal' PSA does not exclude prostate cancer, but the lower the PSA level the less likely the risk.
- In interpreting a PSA result, other causes of raised PSA must be considered (see Table 5.1).
- Misleading PSA results will occur during or shortly after an episode of prostatitis or urinary infection, or following prostatic biopsy or urethral instrumentation.
- In uncertain cases, the possibility of asymptomatic prostatic infection should be considered by treating with antibiotics and then repeating PSA measurement.

In management of prostate cancer
- PSA is a reliable guide to stage of disease, of progression and of response to treatment.
- Inappropriate increase in PSA may occur temporarily in men treated with radiotherapy.
- Occasionally PSA will not predict relapse after hormonal treatment.
- Except to confirm a change, it is unnecessary to monitor PSA at intervals shorter than 3 months.

In diagnosing prostate cancer
- PSA should not be measured without the patient's knowledge.
- In an asymptomatic man, PSA should only be measured after he has been provided with full information about the limitations of the test, the implications of an abnormal result, the risks of, and false-

negative results from, prostatic biopsy and the uncertainty surrounding treatment of early prostate cancer.

- PSA testing is appropriate in the man with lower urinary symptoms, but information should be provided to allow him to 'opt out' if he wishes.
- Unless prostate cancer is suspected clinically, PSA should only be measured in men who may benefit from curative treatment of early disease; in general those with a life expectation of >10 years and without significant co-morbidity.
- In cases of suspected prostate cancer, the result should be interpreted in the light of the indication. Metastatic disease is unusual with a PSA <10 and unlikely <20 (usually it will be >100).
- Specificity is increased by considering the age-related range (see Table 5.2). The PSA level is related to prostate size – a modest elevation gives more concern if the prostate is small. A rapid increase in serial (3-monthly) measurements increases the suspicion of cancer.
- Measurements of free to total or complexed PSA increase discrimination but are currently only appropriate in secondary care.
- Different methods of PSA measurement may not give equivalent numerical results and different levels than those quoted in the literature may apply.
- Guidance should be accepted from the local Clinical Biochemistry Department.
- Care is necessary in interpreting serial results if measurements come from more than one laboratory.
- If a laboratory changes its method, a period of adjustment will be necessary – dual assays may be provided during the changeover, but care should be taken before ascribing significance to a change in numerical value during this time.

PSA – an introduction

The introduction of PSA has revolutionized the management of prostate cancer, yet no topic is more controversial. Its importance justifies a whole section to itself.

PSA: its nature and significance

In its role in reproduction, the prostate produces a number of organ-specific substances. As described on p. 8 ('Function of the prostate'), PSA, a protease glycoprotein enzyme of molecular mass 39 kDa, is a normal component of seminal plasma. In the blood, it is inactivated by binding (complexed – cPSA) to proteins, most to α1-antichymotrypsin (ACT) and some to α2-macroglobulin (α2M) (Figure 5.1). Some inactive PSA circulates in an unbound form. The standard PSA measurements detected a mixture of complexed and free PSA; 'total PSA' assays may well underestimate the true amount of PSA in the serum. While the 'free PSA' is heterogenous in origin, an important component, BPSA, seems to be produced predominantly from benign prostatic hyperplasia (BPH) tissue. Selective measurements of these 'isoforms' of PSA might increase specificity of PSA as a diagnostic test.

PSA, then, is produced selectively by the prostate, but *not* specifically by prostate cancer. Indeed, a cancer cell actually produces less PSA than does a 'benign' one. The amount of PSA in the serum is dependent on the size of the prostate but also on the integrity of the 'barrier' between prostate and serum, which determines, for a given size of gland, the serum PSA level. While the disruption of the prostatic architecture within the cancer increases the serum PSA in malignancy, this is but one of the causes of abnormal PSA levels (Table 5.1). These alternative possibilities should always be remembered before jumping to the conclusion that a raised PSA equals prostate cancer. If one of these conditions is known to be present, it should be treated or allowed to resolve before measuring PSA. Note particularly that it can take several months for PSA to return to its 'normal' levels following an episode of acute prostatitis (see Chapter 19).

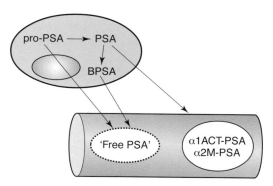

Figure 5.1   PSA in serum: free and complexed PSA. ACT, α1-antichymotrypsin; α2M, α2-macroglobulin.

Table 5.1 Causes of elevation of serum PSA

Benign prostatic enlargement
Infection of urinary tract (especially acute prostatitis – see Chapter 19)
Prostatic surgery and urethral instrumentation (including catheterization)
Prostatic biopsy
Ejaculation
Bicycle riding
Prostate cancer

Note that diagnostic digital rectal examination (DRE) of the prostate will not affect PSA levels, although vigorous prostatic massage might have some effect.

PSA methodology

It will be noticed that there is some vagueness in this section about numerical PSA levels. This is partly because the various methods used to measure PSA have ranges that do not always coincide. With improved quality control this may become less of a problem in future, but it is important to accept guidance about reference ranges from the local laboratory. The differences are fairly small and mainly a problem in patients whose PSA is being sequentially monitored. Caution is particularly needed in two circumstances:

- when the care of a patient is shared between primary care and a specialist who would normally use different biochemistry laboratories;
- when the laboratory changes its method.

In the latter case, the laboratory will probably cover the transition by making dual assays, but there may be confusion when a patient has two measurements spanning the transition, but a long time apart.

PSA in the management of prostate cancer (see Chapters 12–16)

Whatever the controversy and difficulty surrounding PSA as a diagnostic and screening test, PSA has indubitably revolutionized the management of the disease, once diagnosed. Serum PSA levels reflect the tumour load and stage (Figure 5.2), increase with disease progression and fall as a result of successful treatment (Figure 5.3).

30

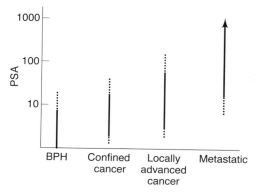

Figure 5.2 Ranges of PSA levels in benign and malignant disease.

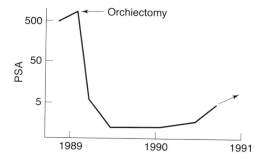

Figure 5.3 Response of PSA to treatment of metastatic prostate cancer in one patient. PSA rose on disease recurrence; patient asymptomatic at time of last PSA measurement, but developed spinal cord compression within 2 months.

Staging information

Each stage of the disease has a characteristic range of PSA associated with it, albeit ones which overlap each other and that of BPH (see Figure 5.2). Thus, it is unlikely that a man with metastatic disease will have a PSA of less than 10, and indeed his PSA is likely to be in three figures. This is important, for example, when investigating back pain of uncertain origin. While a PSA of 9 might mean that he does have prostate cancer, it is most unlikely that it will have metastasized and thus is not the cause of his back pain. It also means that in assessing men for radical treatment, bone scans are often omitted if the PSA is less than 10.

Disease progression

Where, for whatever reason, expectant management is selected, PSA is the principal method of assessing disease progression. It is usual, in the initial stages, to measure PSA at 3-monthly intervals. Indeed, unless to confirm an unexpected change in level, there are few circumstances in which more frequent measurements are needed. It is the nature of cancer to progress, so it is to be expected that PSA will increase. The purpose of monitoring is to identify rapidly developing disease at a stage when treatment will still be effective. Although it is difficult to give rigid rules, if the rate of increase is such that the PSA would double in less than 2 years, it is likely that the disease is aggressive. It is important to remember that the alternative causes of PSA elevation still can occur even in men with cancer, and increases, particularly if unexpected or particularly sharp, should be confirmed by a repeat measurement before treatment is started or changed. PSA results should not be followed slavishly, and always considered in a clinical context. If worrying non-specific symptoms occur, a stable PSA can be reassuring that they are not related to the cancer.

Response to treatment

Monitoring PSA is now the main method of follow-up at all stages of the disease. The rate and extent of the decrease in PSA following treatment has prognostic significance (see p. 114, 'PSA in follow-up').

Reliability of PSA

While there are few investigations in oncology as useful as PSA, there are some pitfalls.

- A few prostate cancers do not express usual levels of PSA; often these are aggressive, poorly differentiated tumours.
- Following radical prostatectomy, sometimes a very low PSA level persists without evidence of residual disease. It is now recognized that small amounts of benign prostatic tissue left at the bladder neck or urethral margin can account for this.
- After radiotherapy, following a therapeutic fall to the post-treatment nadir, a transient rise may occur, without evidence of disease progression, with subsequent return to the nadir level.

- Following hormone treatment, relapse can occur with little or no increase in PSA, and indeed, even when PSA does rise, it rarely returns to pre-treatment levels.

As with any test, PSA results have to be interpreted in the light of clinical assessment. It has not superseded all other investigations. For example, in a man with bone metastases, alkaline phosphatase may be as useful a marker of progression following treatment as will be the PSA.

PSA as a diagnostic or screening test

Although general practitioners may well share the care of men with prostate cancer, and monitor their PSA in association with the urologist or oncologist (see p. 114, 'PSA in follow-up'), it is in the controversial areas of diagnosis and screening that PSA has most impact in primary care. Enthusiastic publicity in the media and vigorous advocacy by support groups contrasts with the coolness of the authorities. Differences in opinion among the 'experts' must leave the general practitioner greeted by a request for 'a test for prostate cancer' from one of his patients feeling confused.

On the one hand, while advanced prostate cancer is incurable, PSA can identify it at an early stage, enabling it to be cured by radical prostatectomy. Since early prostate cancer is usually asymptomatic, it might seem logical to recommend that men over 50 should undergo regular PSA tests. However, PSA is a non-specific test, and the majority of men with a mild elevation will not have prostate cancer. Prostate cancer curable by radical surgery has a good prognosis and any benefit from this intervention will not occur for many years. Invasive treatment with significant side effects is unnecessary for many, as they will die from other diseases before their prostate cancer becomes fatal. There is no definite evidence that PSA testing will save lives and hence at present there is a tendency to discourage its use as a 'screening procedure'. It is worth noting that even in the USA where a substantial proportion of men undergo regular PSA tests, population screening for prostate cancer is not public policy.

Specificity of PSA in diagnosing cancer

An elevation of PSA above normal levels can be due to a variety of causes (see Table 5.1). It is important particularly to recognize the effect of infection. In cases of infection, it is essential that the infection is eradicated and then several weeks left until a meaningful measurement can be made. Asymptomatic prostatitis (see Chapter 19) can also cause a spuriously raised PSA, and sometimes a 4-week course of a quinolone antibiotic will return an unexplained PSA level to normal. Similarly, PSA should not be measured after biopsy (when it may be elevated for several weeks) or urethral instrumentation – also catheterization, a source of diagnostic difficulty in men with retention of urine. When an unexpectedly high result occurs, enquiry about ejaculation and bicycle riding may reveal the true cause. Indeed, it is worth advising a few days' abstinence from these activities (for both there seems to be no upper age limit!) when arranging the test.

These aspects aside, the overlap in PSA levels between benign hyperplasia and early cancer (Figure 5.2) is the main reason for the lack of specificity in cancer diagnosis. Although the higher the PSA, the greater the chance of cancer (Table 5.2), unfortunately, at those PSA levels that will confidently predict cancer, it is likely that the disease will be too advanced for curative treatment. In the 'grey area' when PSA is less than 10, approximately a third of men will have cancer, which can only be confirmed by biopsy. If this were a safe and reliable procedure, this would not be an issue (see p. 87, 'Biopsy'), but serious complications still occur. Despite improvements in biopsy technique which have increased its sensitivity, a proportion of cancers will not be diagnosed. This means that it is difficult easily to reassure a man that his elevated PSA is not due to cancer, and in many cases repeat biopsy is needed. If he has had problems with the first biopsy he may be reluctant to repeat the experience, yet remain worried about his possible cancer. Thus it is essential that a man be informed of these issues before a PSA test is done (see p. 36, 'Opportunist screening').

Table 5.2 Relation of serum PSA level to risk of prostate cancer

PSA	Risk of prostate cancer
<4.0	Found in 20% of men with prostate cancer
4–10	25–30% will have prostate cancer
>10	>60% will have prostate cancer

Improving the specificity of PSA testing – PSA density and velocity

Avoiding or reversing alternative causes of PSA elevation, or appreciating that they might have occurred, is clearly essential, and in particular, reassurance to the patient that this is a possibility may prevent a period of undue anxiety.

The level of PSA in BPH is related to the size of the gland and in BPH any increase in PSA will be far slower than if it were due to progressing prostate cancer. To distinguish between BPH and cancer as a cause of 'raised' PSA, the concepts of prostate specific acid density (PSAD) and of velocity (PSAV) or PSA doubling time have been developed. Although attempts to formalize these into discriminatory numerical ranges have not been successful, they are useful concepts. A PSA of, say, 8 is of far less concern in a man with a huge benign-feeling prostate than if his prostate is barely enlarged. Similarly a PSA which increases rapidly over a few months demands more aggressive investigation (including repeated biopsy) than one which is stable. A low PSA doubling time also suggests that, even if an undisclosed cancer were present, it is unlikely to be aggressive.

Age-related PSA

PSA rises with increasing age, mainly as a result of age-related prostatic enlargement. This is the basis of the age-related PSA range (Table 5.3). This is an important concept; the quoted normal range of 0–4 (for most methods in use – see p. 30, 'PSA methodology') will mask a PSA which for a young man may well be consistent with possible cancer. Using the higher range for the older man will avoid necessary concern and intrusive investigation. It also, incidentally, directs the investigation of raised PSA towards the younger man, who has most to gain from diagnosis of early

Table 5.3   Age-related PSA levels

Age (years)	PSA cut-off (ng/l)
50–59	≥3.0
60–69	≥4.0
≥70	>5.0

prostate cancer. Increasingly, Clinical Biochemistry Departments will report age-related ranges for PSA.

PSA isoforms

As described earlier (Figure 5.1), part of the circulating PSA is in an inactive unbound form, a component of which is produced predominantly from BPH tissue. Thus, if a 'raised' PSA results from benign enlargement, a larger proportion of this PSA will be in the unbound ('free') form and the ratio of free to total PSA (f/tPSA) will be higher (>20%, exact cut-off depending on the method). This can be assessed either by a measurement of f/tPSA, or by selectively measuring the bound or 'complexed' PSA (cPSA). At present these measurements have not replaced total PSA as the first-line test, and are mainly appropriate for use in secondary care. A high f/tPSA is certainly reassuring when prostatic biopsy has not diagnosed cancer.

Screening for prostate cancer

Does the existence of a simple blood test which can identify a group of men at risk of having prostate cancer provide a basis for cancer screening? As demonstrated in this chapter, the interpretation of a raised PSA is far from simple, and even if prostate cancer is diagnosed, there remains considerable debate on how it should be managed. There is at present insufficient evidence to institute a screening programme similar to that for breast and cervical cancer. It is important to emphasize that this statement is based as much on scientific as on economic considerations.

Opportunist screening

Many men will seek a PSA test. With increasing emphasis on preventative medicine, and as regular health checks, whether in NHS primary care or in the private sector, have become more popular, should PSA become part of routine health screening? Why not check the PSA when he is in for his blood pressure recording, or having a regular cholesterol measurement? Publicity about cancer in general repeatedly emphasizes the need for early diagnosis and treatment, against which it is difficult to argue. However, prostate cancer is not like other cancers. Many men with the disease do not need immediate treatment; many will never need it. Even where a man needs treatment for early cancer, it represents a considerable investment in immediate discomfort and potential morbidity to forestall a disease process which may have no adverse effects for many years. Diagnosis, despite the strides made in the last decade, remains imprecise. To do a PSA test without prior discussion with the patient could be seen as an abdication of a doctor's responsibility.

It is now accepted good practice that in the absence of a clinical indication, PSA is only measured if the patient has been fully informed of the issues. Information sheets (for example, Appendix 1) are available to inform him of the issues, and BUPA and other organizations with health screening programmes do this.

Men with LUTS

Although not universally accepted as good practice, most prostate assessment clinics (PACs) include PSA testing as part of their protocols. However, this should not prevent the patient being acquainted with the issues, although here it is more a matter of his opting out than opting in.

6 PROSTATE DISEASE AND LOWER URINARY SYMPTOMS – CLINICAL ASSESSMENT

Management points

- In assessing lower urinary symptoms (LUTS) in the male, the length of history, reason for consultation, nature and severity of symptoms and the bother they cause are important.
- Severity of symptoms and the bother they cause are assessed by the International Prostate Symptom Score (IPSS) (Figure 6.1). This is a measure of severity of symptoms, not of their aetiology.
- Other symptoms may need exploring. Haematuria requires separate URGENT investigation. Dysuria and abdominal pain may be coincidental. A history of perineal trauma, urethritis or instrumentation may raise the possibility of urethral stricture.
- Symptoms of renal failure may predominate in a man with chronic retention, who may complain of few urinary symptoms.
- Physical examination should include the genitalia to exclude phimosis. Digital rectal examination (DRE) will exclude an obvious advanced carcinoma, but otherwise is unhelpful. The size of the prostate has no bearing on the symptoms, although it might affect choice of treatment.
- Assessment of general condition is important; referral for investigation of possible early prostate cancer, or for surgery for benign prostatic hyperplasia (BPH), may not be appropriate in an elderly man with debilitating co-morbidity.

The history

The man complaining of lower urinary tract symptoms (LUTS) needs careful assessment if appropriate treatment is to be given. The length of history, distinction between storage and voiding symptoms, severity of symptoms

International Prostate Symptom Score (IPSS)	None	Less than 1 time in 5	Less than half the time	About half the time	More than half the time	Almost always	Score
1 Over the past month how often have you had a sensation of not emptying your bladder completely after you finished urinating?	0	1	2	3	4	5	
2 Over the past month how often have you had to urinate again less than two hours after you finished urinating?	0	1	2	3	4	5	
3 Over the past month, how often have you found that you stopped and started again several times when you urinated?	0	1	2	3	4	5	
4 Over the past month how often have you found it difficult to postpone urination?	0	1	2	3	4	5	
5 Over the past month how often have you had a weak urinary stream?	0	1	2	3	4	5	
6 Over the past month how often have you had to push or strain to begin urination	0	1	2	3	4	5	
7 Over the past month how often did you most typically get up to urinate from the time you went to bed at night until the time you get up in the morning?	none	x 1	x 2	x 3	x 4	x 5	
Total IPSS score							

Quality of life due to urinary symptoms

	Delighted	Pleased	Mostly Satisfied	Mixed Feelings	Mostly dissatisfied	Unhappy	Terrible	QoL
If you were to spend the rest of your life with your urinary condition just the way it is now, how would you feel about it?	0	1	2	3	4	5	6	

Figure 6.1 International Prostate Symptom Score (IPSS)

and amount of bother caused are all important. The context in which the symptoms come to light, whether from direct questioning during a consultation for another condition, concern by the patient that comparatively mild symptoms may be due to cancer, or symptoms so severe as to be disabling, is also important in planning appropriate management.

Length of history

Some men have long-standing, if not lifelong, symptoms which may not be reported until middle age. Such symptoms are unlikely to be due to 'the prostate' and the prognosis for successful treatment, particularly of storage symptoms, is poor. On the other hand, a short history has been said to raise suspicion of prostate cancer. In the author's experience this is not necessarily so, as many cancers diagnosed now are coincidental to the benign prostatic hyperplasia (BPH) causing the symptoms (see p. 20, 'Pathology and epidemiology of prostate cancer'). A short history of storage symptoms may be due to recent onset of instability/bladder overactivity in a man who had not appreciated the significance of the much longer period of poor urine flow he had experienced. Prostatitis may cause a sudden deterioration in LUTS without associated dysuria.

Symptom scores

Currently, the International Prostate Symptom Score (IPSS) (Figure 6.1) is most widely used. It gives a numerical indicator of the severity of the symptoms (to a maximum of 35), the individual questions dealing with storage and voiding symptoms. The second element, the 'Bothersome Index', is a crude measure of the effect of the symptoms on the patient's quality of life. The patient is usually asked to complete the IPSS prior to consultation, although it is important to review it with him to ensure the questions have been understood. In interpreting the IPSS score, the following points should be noted:

- International *Prostate* Symptom Score is a misnomer – it is used to measure the severity of the patient's symptoms, not to diagnosis prostate disease. More appropriate would be 'International *Lower Urinary Tract* Symptom Score'. Given to a group of elderly women, a range of scores similar to that recorded by men with prostatic disease would be obtained.

- While 'incomplete bladder emptying' can be due to a high residual urine volume after voiding, it is also a symptom associated with instability even if the bladder is empty. In other words, it can be considered as either a voiding or a storage symptom.
- The individual symptom most likely to be inaccurately scored is the urine flow. The onset of a deteriorating urine flow is often insidious or may be dismissed as 'due to old age' and thus under-scored. It is worthwhile to ask specifically whether his flow is as good as he remembered it 10 years ago, or where he hits the wall in a public urinal, and whether other men come and go while he is using it.
- An adequate flow is only achieved if a reasonable volume of urine is passed. A man with severe storage symptoms may rarely pass a sufficient volume to produce an adequate flow and may give this symptom a misleading high score. Asking if he always has a poor flow or if his flow improves if he does pass a high volume is helpful. Even men with severe nocturia will often wake in the morning with a full bladder. 'How is your flow first thing in the morning?' is a useful question – it is likely to be at its best for the man with storage symptoms but worst when there really is obstruction.
- The 'bothersome index' will not necessarily reflect the symptom score. A man may have a score in single figures, but if he is getting up five times a night even with few other symptoms he will have a poor quality of life. Also, the bothersome index often reflects a man's concern about cancer, and will improve once he is reassured.

Other symptoms

Frank (visible) haematuria almost always requires urgent investigation for potential bladder (or renal) cancer. Dysuria may indicate prostatitis rather than BPH. Except in acute retention, abdominal pain is not a feature of BPH. Erectile dysfunction occurs in the same age group as LUTS due to BPH. Any relationship between them is tenuous but the patient may relate the two, or out of embarrassment use the LUTS as reason for consulting – 'while I'm here …'.

One important, although uncommon, presentation of prostate disease is renal failure due to high-pressure chronic retention, which is important because, unlike most causes of renal failure at this age, it is curable. The symptoms themselves may be non-specific (loss of appetite, nausea, symptoms of anaemia, etc.). The patient may complain of few, if any, urinary symptoms. Abdominal examination will usually reveal a distended bladder.

Past history

As urethral stricture is an important differential diagnosis, urologists are interested in any history of trauma, urethritis (chlamydial infection, gonorrhoea) or instrumentation. Operations where catheterization is routine, particularly cardiac surgery, are especially relevant. Previous prostate operations can also cause strictures; also, BPH can recur, so a previous transurethral resection of the prostate (TURP), even if initially successful, will not preclude recurrent bladder outflow obstruction (BOO).

Physical examination

In the primary care setting this may not contribute much. Abdominal examination may reveal a distended bladder (sometimes difficult in an obese man). It is worth examining the foreskin as a tight phimosis can cause similar symptoms to BOO.

Digital rectal examination (DRE)

In primary care, the value of a DRE (an abbreviation which has replaced 'PR') is limited and indeed in some guidelines and pathways it is omitted. It is true that early prostate cancer is often not palpable, and that detecting the more subtle changes of early prostate cancer does perhaps require the experience of a specialist. However, a grossly malignant, hard irregular prostate might affect the urgency with which a referral is made, especially if (for example, in an elderly man) the PSA would not otherwise have been measured (see p. 36, 'Opportunistic screening'). Estimating the size of the benign prostate is less important. Size really only impinges on management, usually a matter for the urologist. Although it is a factor in suitability for treatment with a 5α-reductase inhibitor (see p. 58, 'Medical treatment of BPH'), PSA is a more reliable surrogate for this purpose. Increasingly, specialist nurse practitioners running prostate assessment clinics (PACs) are being trained in DRE. As they will often see a dozen or more patients a week, they will rapidly gain an expertise not available to someone who only has occasional need for this skill.

It is perhaps unnecessary to record that this is a *rectal* examination. However, an examination focused solely on the prostate might overlook a coincidental rectal carcinoma on the posterior wall – at best a source of embarrassment when it caused symptoms later!

Overall assessment of the patient

In primary care, the patient's full medical history is available and he will often have been known for many years. The importance of his symptoms, the significance of a diagnosis and the appropriateness of potentially invasive treatments all interact on management decisions, a process which should start in the primary care consulting room. Raising the possibility of early prostate cancer with an 80-year-old man with severe cardio-respiratory disease could be a source of distress without possibility of benefit. Most urologists are happy to discuss whether an individual patient requires referral, for which there may also be local guidelines.

7 INVESTIGATION OF PROSTATIC DISEASE

Management points

- Investigation is needed to confirm the presence of obstruction and its severity, and to exclude other causes for lower urinary tract symptoms (LUTS). The following are appropriate in primary care.

Laboratory tests

- Urinalysis and, if abnormal, culture. This excludes infection, may indicate a cystoscopy to exclude bladder tumour or stones if there is haematuria. Glycosuria indicating diabetes may come to light as a cause of frequency (polyuria).
- Serum creatinine.
- PSA is to be measured according to the guidance in Chapter 5.
- Full blood count, only necessary if there is haematuria or poor renal function.

Bladder function tests

- Increasingly available via open access to a Flow Clinic or Prostate Assessment Clinic (PAC) in local urology department.
- Flow rate >20 excludes significant obstruction, <8 indicates severe obstruction – but can occur with atonic/weak detrusor muscle without actual obstruction.
- A voided volume >150 ml is needed for an accurate flow measurement.
- Residual urine (RU), which can be measured by simple ultrasound device. Small or no RU does not exclude obstruction. RU >500 ml merits referral.
- Both flow rate and RU measurements are more reliable on repetition.

Investigation in secondary care

- Cystoscopy is indicated to exclude suspected urethral stricture, and bladder cancer, which may present with storage symptoms (especially when associated with frank or occult haematuria).

- **Urodynamics: filling cystometrogram will diagnose bladder instability; voiding cystometrogam is the only reliable method of confirming obstruction and is advisable before surgery for benign prostatic hyperplasia (BPH).**
- **Imaging is only needed in selected cases: ultrasound scan of kidneys if renal function poor; imaging of upper tracts (IVU, ultrasound or CT) in patients with haematuria.**

Investigation of the patient with LUTS

This is needed to:

- confirm the aetiology of the symptoms – whether due to bladder outflow obstruction (BOO) or from other causes;
- differentiate between potential causes of obstruction. This includes exclusion of carcinoma of the prostate, whether it be advanced disease actually causing lower urinary tract symptoms (LUTS) or a coincidental tumour. In the latter case, consider the advice on PSA testing in Chapter 5;
- assess severity of obstruction, which in turn determines the appropriate treatment.

Although it is difficult in practice to separate the issue of cancer of the prostate, this will be dealt with in the relevant chapters and here the concern is mainly the man with symptoms possibly due to benign prostatic hyperplasia (BPH).

An indication of the possible aetiology and severity of the symptoms will already have been obtained from the history and examination. Investigation involves in all cases functional tests, and in selected patients, imaging and endoscopy. The days in which any man with lower urinary symptoms routinely underwent an intravenous urogram (IVU) are long past and imagining (other than to assess residual urine volumes) has only a minor role.

Laboratory investigations

Urinalysis and culture
Urinalysis is appropriate – as discussed elsewhere, storage symptoms can be a presentation of bladder tumour and the need for a cystoscopy is

reinforced if there is blood in the urine. Note that haematuria is not a predictor of prostate cancer and for most urologists would not affect the decision whether to measure the PSA. Urinalysis will also pick up glycosuria in men with diabetes presenting with polyuria. The typical symptoms of bladder outflow obstruction are unlikely to be due to urinary infection, and urine culture is only really indicated when there is dysuria or other symptoms suggestive of infection, or abnormality on urinalysis.

Serum biochemistry
It is logical to measure serum creatinine, bearing in mind that renal failure due to bladder outflow obstruction is normally a complication of chronic retention. In most cases, the other tests in the routine 'biochemical profile' will provide little useful information.

Prostate specific antigen (PSA)
This has been dealt with in Chapter 5. Suffice to say here that in a man with LUTS, a case can be made for measuring PSA, provided that he is informed it is being done and given sufficient information to 'opt out' if he wishes. In the absence of clinical suspicion of prostate cancer, measurement of PSA is unlikely to be useful in someone with limited life expectation, whether due to age or to co-morbidity. PSA does have a role in identifying men who will benefit from 5α-reductase inhibitor treatment (see p. 58, 'Medical treatment of BPH').

Haematology
There is no specific reason to measure a full blood count unless there are other indications, e.g. gross haematuria, clinical suspicion of anaemia, or renal failure.

Bladder function tests

The mainstay of investigation of LUTS is measurement of urine flow rate and residual bladder volume. Flowmeters and bladder scanners are standard equipment in urology clinics and could be used in primary care. Some years ago, the author predicted that urinary flowmeters would become as common in primary care health centres as ECG machines and respiratory peak-flowmeters; a prediction which has yet to be fulfilled.

A more realistic solution is to call on the expertise of the local urology department. Many urology departments have 'flow clinics' and flow rate measurements are an integral part of prostate assessment clinic protocols. Direct access to these facilities from Primary Care is to be encouraged; thus a description of the procedure is appropriate for this book.

Urine flow measurements (Figure 7.1)

The standard flowmeter consists of a funnel into which the patient is asked to pass urine normally, without straining. Most machines start to record automatically, giving a paper readout of the flow curve, and automatically providing a number of numerical values, of which the most important are the peak flow (Q_{max}), and the voided volume.

The hallmark of obstruction is a reduction in urine flow rate:

- A peak flow rate (Q_{max}) in excess of 20 ml/s effectively rules out obstruction.
- A flow below 15 ml/s is consistent with early obstruction.
- One below 8 ml/s suggests significant obstruction, for which surgery may be appropriate.

An optimal flow rate requires the bladder to be adequately filled, with a voided volume of at least 150 ml. Otherwise, the recorded flow rate will be too low. Normograms are available to assist with this problem, and inspection of the actual flow tracing is useful – the curve will preserve its shape but with a lower peak (Figure 7.1b).

The measured flow rate is dependent on both bladder pressure and outflow resistance. Thus a reduced flow rate can be due to weakness of the detrusor muscle without obstruction, and a high voiding pressure can compensate for obstruction.

The voided volume is not only useful in ensuring an accurate Q_{max}. Small volumes consistently obtained after several attempts suggest either instability or a small bladder volume; volumes greater than 500 ml, an over-capacious bladder (Figure 7.1d).

Residual urine

An ultrasound probe is used to identify the bladder and automatically gives a volume recording. Conveniently measured immediately following the flow rate recording, as with that test, care also needs to be taken in interpretation.

50

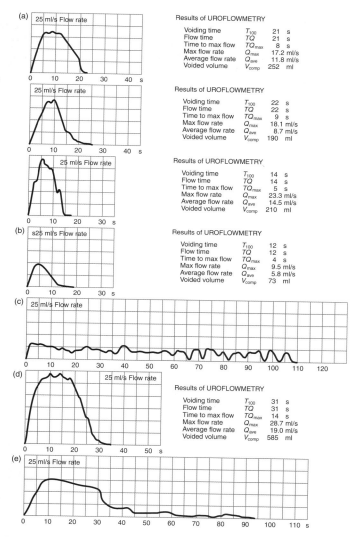

Figure 7.1 Urinary flow records. (a) Examples of normal flow for a man (women's flow rates are higher). (b) Low voided volume without obstruction; flow rate reduced but shape of curve similar to (a). (c) Typical flow record in case of bladder outflow obstruction. (d) Excessive voided volume, indicating abnormal bladder volume. (e) Flow curve in case of urethral stricture. Note typical 'flat top' to curve (compare to c).

- Repeated recordings are useful, with the lowest reading taken as the true value.
- In the past, a residual urine of >200 ml was considered an indication for surgery. This is no longer interpreted as rigidly, but obstruction causing a high residual urine probably does predispose to retention.
- A consistent residual of >500 ml in the absence of pain indicates chronic retention.

Further investigation

The tests described so far are appropriate in almost all cases, and should be accessible to the primary care team. Further investigations, usually only available in the urology department, are needed in specific circumstances.

Cystoscopy

Nowadays a flexible cystoscopy is usually performed under local (topical urethral) anaesthetic. The main indications are:

- the possibility of a urethral stricture, deduced from a history of risk factors (trauma, urethritis, instrumentation/catheterization), symptoms in a young patient, and a characteristic flat topped flow curve (Figure 7.1e);
- to exclude bladder pathology, especially a tumour, as a cause of storage symptoms, particularly with 'dipstick' haematuria.
- Although the prostate is examined during the procedure, its appearance alone is not sufficient to diagnose obstruction. However, its appearance does help to gauge its size, and is sometimes helpful in planning treatment.

Urodynamics

A reduced flow may result from detrusor muscle weakness, and is not diagnostic of BOO. Also, in the presence of severe frequency, an adequate flow measurement is difficult – is the flow poor because of the frequency, or is the frequency secondary to obstruction? The only reliable way to assess obstruction is by urodynamic assessment, which many urologists now consider mandatory before advising surgery for BPH.

The investigation takes place in two phases, a *filling cystometrogram* to assess bladder function, particularly whether there is instability, and a voiding *pressure flow* study to diagnose obstruction. A pressure transducer and a catheter for filling with fluid are passed into the bladder. A transducer is also used to measure rectal pressure, as an indicator of intra-abdominal pressure. Pressure measurements are made both as the bladder fills and during voiding. Spikes of increased pressure during filling indicate instability/overactivity. The relationship between flow rate and pressure in the bladder during voiding indicates whether there is obstruction.

Limitations

As an absolute diagnostic test, standard urodynamics is imprecise, with many results falling in the equivocal range. The intrusion of catheter and transducer interferes with the normal function. In the standard technique, the bladder is filled more rapidly than the rate of physiological urine secretion. 'Slow filling' urodynamics attempts to reproduce physiological bladder filling, but this is incompatible with the volume of work going through a routine urology department's urodynamic room. 'Ambulatory urodynamics', where a transducer alone is introduced and the pressure measured on a portable device as the patient goes about his usual activities, is one step further, but only available in specialized centres.

Imaging

Other than to measure residual urine, imaging now plays only a minor role in assessment of the man with BPH.

- An ultrasound scan of the kidneys may be indicated to exclude hydronephrosis if renal function is abnormal.
- If a bladder stone is suspected, a plain x-ray or ultrasound scan of the bladder may be ordered.
- Urethral stricture will be diagnosed by flexible cystoscopy; urethrograms are mainly indicated in planning treatment of the stricture.
- The only indication for an intravenous urogram (IVU) is in cases of haematuria (although increasingly replaced by ultrasound or CT) or (coincidental) suspected ureteric calculi.

- Transrectal ultrasound to image the prostate is essentially an investigation for suspected prostate cancer, although it can be used to obtain an accurate measurement of prostatic size.

8 MANAGEMENT OF MEN WITH LOWER URINARY SYMPTOMS IN PRIMARY CARE

Management points

- This section deals with lower urinary symptoms resulting from benign enlargement. Diagnosis of prostate cancer and its management are dealt with in Chapters 5 and 12 *et seq.*
- The International Prostate Symptom Score (IPSS) is a measure of the nature and severity of the symptoms, and how troublesome they are ('bothersome index')
- Mild symptoms (IPSS <7) may not need treatment. Consultation is often due to worry about cancer.
- Measurement of PSA (after providing appropriate information) with digital rectal examination (DRE) can resolve cancer worries.
- A normal flow rate and residual urine accurately excludes bladder outflow obstruction (BOO). These results can be determined by direct referral to a hospital Flow Clinic or Prostate Assessment Clinic (PAC). If these investigations are normal, and symptoms themselves do not merit treatment, no further action, nor consultant referral, is necessary.
- Moderate symptoms (IPSS 7–19) usually are treated medically and can be managed in primary care. Two classes of drugs are used – $\alpha 1$-adrenergic antagonists (α-blockers), e.g. alfuzosin and tamsulosin, and 5α-reductase inhibitors, finasteride and dutasteride.
- α-Adrenergic antagonist drugs work rapidly and are the treatment of choice where the prostate is not significantly enlarged and for bothersome symptoms.
- 5α-Reductase inhibitors (finasteride, dutasteride) reduce the prostate size and will only benefit men with significant enlargement.
- PSA >1.4 can be used as a surrogate for suitablilty for 5α-reductase treatment.

55

- 5α-Reductase inhibitors reduce PSA levels by 50% – any concern about 'raised' PSA should be resolved before starting treatment.
- Evidence in favour of combination treatment is provided by recent clinical trials.
- Risk of retention can be reduced by 5α-reductase inhibitor treatment, for which large prostate size is a risk factor.
- Combination treatment may be appropriate if the patient also has severely bothersome symptoms.
- While treatment ideally should be initiated following flow and residual urine measurements, a therapeutic trial of medical treatment may be appropriate where these are not available.
- With mild and moderate symptoms, lifestyle advice, particularly regarding fluid intake, should be given in addition to any pharmaceutical treatment.
- Open access referral to a PAC where available locally may provide the most effective method of assessing men with mild or moderate symptoms.
- Patients with severe symptoms (IPSS >20), poor flow rates (<8 ml/s) and atypical symptoms require referral according to the algorithms in Chapter 9.
- Herbal remedies are popular; it is important to know if a patient is using one.

Lower urinary symptoms and BPH

This chapter deals essentially with managing lower urinary tract symptoms (LUTS) due to benign disease. Initial management cannot be divorced from concern, and reassurance about possible cancer will be an important issue (see Chapters 5 and 12). However, concern about cancer must not override the importance of benign prostatic hyperplasia (BPH) as a source of LUTS.

The optimum management depends on:

- the severity of the symptoms;
- the confirmation of bladder outflow obstruction, and its severity;
- the needs and the aspirations of the patient;
- assessment of the risk of future complications (e.g. retention of urine).

The International Prostate Symptom Score (IPSS) questionnaire will identify those with mild symptoms (IPSS 0–7) for whom, perhaps, reassurance only may be necessary, and those with such severe symptoms (IPSS >20) that it is unlikely that treatments available in primary care will provide a solution. The intermediate group are those for whom a trial of medical treatment is appropriate, with possibilities for management in primary care. These should be treated as a guide, recognizing that individual men will vary in their response to symptoms – here the 'bothersome' element of the IPSS is helpful. The general practitioner, who may have known the man for many years, is at a distinct advantage over the urologist, to whom the patient will be a stranger with only a short outpatient consultation available in which to get to know his needs.

'Is it serious, doctor?'

Mild lower urinary symptoms are common. Many a man seeks reassurance that he does not have a serious problem. The possibility of cancer will be in the forefront of his mind, perhaps as a result of a newspaper article, or from the experiences of a friend. His symptoms may be minimal, perhaps one or two episodes of nocturia from time to time, with a symptom score of <5. It should be possible to reassure this man within the primary care sector, avoiding, for patients, an anxious wait for an outpatient appointment, for urologists, a distraction from the patients who do require their services, and for GPs, the satisfaction of a rapid resolution of their patient's problem.

Reassurance for the man with a low symptom score is provided by a normal or near-normal flow rate combined with a negligible residual urine, which has a high specificity for excluding significant bladder outflow obstruction (BOO), and, after due counselling (Chapter 5), a PSA value within his age-related range. In a urology clinic, a digital rectal examination (DRE) would also be performed. DRE normally should have little additional value, but the author does feel a DRE is appropriate when a patient declines a PSA measurement. This will exclude the (admittedly remote) possibility of a clinically obvious locally advanced carcinoma, possibly producing few symptoms, for which treatment would be indicated. This is a personal view which may breach current guidelines.

Use of the Prostate Assessment Clinic (PAC)

Currently, the facilities for investigating LUTS within primary care are limited. Both primary care and hospital consultant services are under increasing pressure. NHS policy is one of moving care wherever possible to the community. The best compromise for the majority of men with LUTS is to make use of the nurse-led services available in most urology departments. How these services are used will depend on local practice, for which protocols may be in place. While the primary care team may prefer transmission of the raw data for their own use, in many PACs, the nurse specialist, working to a protocol, will be able to issue the results along with a treatment recommendation, possibly following review of the results by a urologist.

Medical treatment of BPH

Where the symptom score and bothersome index merit treatment, but not surgery, drug therapy is appropriate. Since the improvement in obstruction on medical treatment is limited, patients with flow rates <8 are likely not to benefit that much, but as drug treatment is reversible, a therapeutic trial in primary care is unlikely to cause harm. The exception is the man who has experienced transient retention or episodes of severe hesitancy; he is likely to need surgery to pre-empt acute retention.

Two classes of drugs mainly are used to treat BPH: α1-adrenergic antagonists and 5α-reductase inhibitors.

α1-Adrenergic antagonists ('α-blockers')

The rationale for the use of α-blockers is that the tension in the smooth muscle of the bladder neck and prostatic stroma contributes to outflow obstruction. α-Blocking drugs are also used for hypertension, and two of these, terazosin and doxazosin, are also licensed for use in BOO due to BPH. These drugs do have the side effect of postural hypotension, hence the need to titrate the dose. Occasionally the one drug can be used to treat both conditions in the same patient. So-called selective α-blockers (tamsulosin and alfuzosin) utilize differences between the receptors in the prostate and vascular smooth muscle and are less likely to cause hypotension. Older drugs, prazosin and indoramin, have largely been superseded. α-Blockers may cause retrograde ejaculation. Other side effects include drowsiness, hypotension, syncope, asthenia, depression and headache.

5α-Reductase inhibitors

These drugs (finasteride and dutasteride) block the conversion of testosterone to dihydrotestosterone, the form active in the prostate, but not in most other androgen-dependent target organs. This provides a mechanism for selective androgen deprivation to the prostate. Men who have a rare congenital deficiency of this enzyme do not develop BPH. Administration of 5α-reductase inhibitors when BPH has already occurred shrinks the enlarged prostate, with a modest improvement in symptoms and flow rate. It is a prerequisite that the prostate is actually enlarged for this type of drug to work and the larger the gland, the greater the likely benefit. The other difference from α-blockers is the speed of action; as it takes some time for the gland to shrink, improvement in symptoms usually occurs over a period of 3 or more months, and patients must be warned to persevere with treatment. If treatment is stopped, the prostate will enlarge once more and symptoms will usually recur. Side effects are few, the most common being erectile dysfunction in up to 5% of men, which is usually reversible on stopping the drug. The reduction in prostate volume is associated with a proportional fall in PSA. This did cause concern as possibly masking prostate cancer. In fact, the fall in PSA level is a fairly predictable 50%, and once it has stabilized at this level, PSA can be monitored, in the usual way, provided the patient remains on the drug. PSA only becomes a problem if the drug is taken intermittently, which is therapeutically inappropriate.

Prevention of complications from BPH
Can the use of medical treatment prevent later complications? Clinical trials have suggested this to be the case. In particular, finasteride has been shown to reduce both the incidence of acute retention and the need for future surgical treatment by 50%. It must be emphasized that these complications were experienced by only a minority of patients in the trials and the absolute risk reduction was small. Routine use of drugs purely for prophylaxis against retention is probably not appropriate. It is worth considering in men particularly at risk – those with large prostates (for which 5α-reductase inhibitors are most effective anyway), who have low flow rates and high residual urine.

Combined treatment
Since these two classes of drugs act in different ways, would there be an advantage in their combination? Clinical trial has shown an additive effect, but this will, of course, be at increased cost, both in terms of potential side effects and expense.

Choice of medical treatment

α-Blockers are perhaps the first choice for a therapeutic trial in primary care. As their onset is rapid, they are ideal for the man severely bothered by his symptoms. Being readily reversible, they will not interfere with subsequent investigation if treatment is unsuccessful. They are, however, more prone to side effects.

5α-Reductase inhibitors do not rapidly reduce symptoms, and are unsuitable for temporary treatment while a man is awaiting investigation, as any conflicting effects (including the reduction of PSA) are only slowly reversible. They are inappropriate when the prostate is small; then α-blockers are really the only option. Even for a urologist, assessment of the real size of the prostate on DRE can be difficult, and in this context, a PSA >1.4 can be used as a surrogate indication for 5α-reductase inhibitor treatment. The issues surrounding PSA measurement discussed in Chapter 5 do still apply, particularly since the man with the very large prostate most suitable for this treatment may well, simply by virtue of this, have a PSA above the age-related range. It is when there is a large prostate, associated with a low flow and large residual urine, that the risk of future acute retention may indicate treatment even if not merited by symptoms alone.

Combined treatment

If there are severe symptoms combined with risk factors for retention, the patient may wish for some relief from his symptoms without waiting 3 months for the 5α-reductase inhibitor to take effect. A compromise here is to discontinue the α-blocker after, say, 6 months, unless on doing so, the symptoms deteriorate once more.

Other drugs used to treat lower urinary symptoms

Anticholinergic drugs

These drugs (e.g. oxybutynin, tolterodine) used to treat storage symptoms in both sexes, familiar in primary care, do have a role in the management of elderly men with LUTS. When investigation has ruled out obstruction, they would be the treatment of choice in primary instability/overactivity. When there is obstruction, the theoretical risk that reducing bladder contractility might tip the patient into retention probably is small, although the author would be reluctant to use them in a man with a large residual urine or very poor flow. There is no real reason why they cannot be used in conjunction with α-blockers or 5α-reductase inhibitors when storage symptoms persist, and they have a clear role for the man whose bladder instability does not respond to surgery.

Phytotherapy and other 'natural remedies'

Many remedies are advertised for 'prostate health' or for treatment of BPH or cancer. There is little doubt than some of these do contain agents with pharmacological effects, perhaps as antiandrogens, or weak 5α-reductase inhibitors. It is often difficult to shake the perception that agents of uncertain composition and of variable quality are safer and in some way 'better' than purified conventional drugs, of proven efficacy, whose safety has been extensively investigated in clinical trials.

These substances may well have beneficial effects, and there is no real evidence of harm from their use or of interaction with conventional treatments. There is, however, one note of caution. As hormonal effects are a possible mechanism of action, some drugs (the author believes this to be the case with the popular *Saw Palmetto*) may affect PSA levels. The best advice is to accept that patients *will* take these substances, but to make sure that we are aware when they are used.

9   WHEN TO REFER

Management points

- Patients will be referred either because of suspected prostate cancer (Figure 9.1), because investigations not available in primary care are needed or because symptoms require hospital treatment (Figure 9.2).

Referral with possible prostate cancer is appropriate
- Where there is clinically evident disease.
- In men with 'raised' PSA for whom curative treatment of localized disease is appropriate (life expectation >10 years).

Referral for treatment
- Acute retention (usually emergency admission, but see p. 77, 'Acute retention').
- Chronic retention.
- Severe symptoms (IPSS >20) or obstruction (flow Q_{max} <8 ml/s).
- Bothersome symptoms failing to respond to medical treatment.

Referral for cystoscopy if the following are suspected
- Bladder tumour. This includes men with severe storage symptoms, especially if of recent or sudden onset.
- Urethral stricture.
- Bladder stone.

- The individual circumstances and preferences of the patient may override rigid application of guidelines. Introduction of 'patient choice' may influence referral and complicate application of local protocols.

Despite the increased opportunities for management of prostate disease in primary care, there remain a number of indications for referral to a urologist. Indeed, the role of the primary care team suggested in this volume will better identify these men and enable referral in the most appropriate manner. While referral is essential for diagnosis and management when prostate cancer is suspected, there are equally important referral indications for men with benign disease. Surgical treatment is needed for severe symptoms associated with significant outflow obstruction. Surgery is required either for, or to pre-empt, the major complications of benign obstruction, retention of urine and renal failure. Some urinary symptoms are unlikely to be due to prostatic disease and others have a differential diagnosis that might include bladder cancer or stones, requiring urological investigation, as may other causes of outflow obstruction such as urethral stricture.

When making a referral, it is important to consider the reason for doing so – this may affect its urgency and also enable appropriate use to be made of any fast-track or one-stop services available locally. The urologist will find it helpful to know the circumstances of the referral – the patient who has originally consulted because he is severely bothered by lower urinary symptoms requires a different approach to one who has consulted simply because he is worried about the significance of otherwise minimal symptoms, or when the GP has suggested referral because some urinary symptoms have come to light during a consultation about an unrelated issue.

Does this man have prostate cancer?

Possibly this question should be phrased 'does he need treatment for prostate cancer?' These issues are dealt with in detail in Chapters 5 and 12, but some points are worth re-emphasizing here. In short, the decision to refer and the degree of urgency depends on whether there is clinical evidence or suspicion of prostate cancer, the level of PSA and the patient's age and health (in other words, whether his life expectation is likely to exceed 10 years) – see Figure 9.1. In interpreting a PSA result, it is essential to do so in the light of the indication for measuring it. Thus in a young man whose interest is in diagnosis and treatment of early prostate cancer any PSA level above the age-related range would be significant. On the other hand, in a man of 80, treatment of *early* prostate cancer is not an issue. It would, however, be reasonable to measure his PSA to exclude metastatic prostate cancer as a (treatable) cause of backache. If his PSA was elevated but <10, he might indeed have localized prostate cancer, which for him would be insignificant, but metastatic disease would be extremely unlikely. Another cause should be sought for his backache; referral for investigation of prostate cancer would only cause anxiety with little likelihood of benefit.

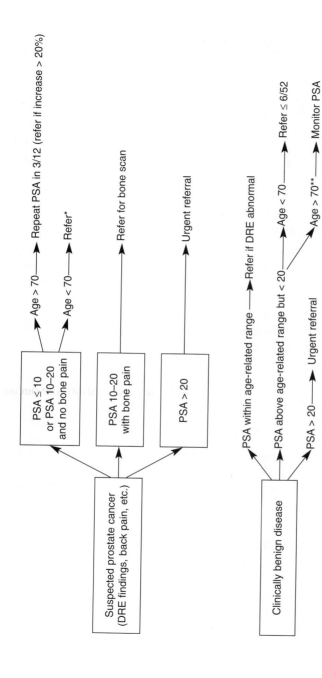

Figure 9.1 Suggested referral pathways for man with possible prostate cancer. *Urgency of referral depends on whether radical treatment for prostate carcinoma would be appropriate – see p. 85, 'Referral'. **PSA measurement not recommended in > 70-year-olds (i.e. men with life expectation < 10 years) unless there is clinical suspicion of prostate carcinoma. Age 70 is a guide only, depending on fitness, co-morbidity, etc.

Referral in benign disease

It is likely that most urology units will have a Prostate Assessment Clinic (PAC) or at least a referral protocol for men with lower urinary symptoms, and local protocols will apply. In some areas, direct access to a PAC will assist in identifying those patients requiring urological intervention, and indeed the PAC protocol will often automatically organize appropriate action. The advice given here should be interpreted in the light of local protocols (which it should not override) and the level of diagnostic services available to the primary care team, whether 'in-house' or by direct access to hospital facilities.

Retention of urine

Painful *acute retention* conventionally is an emergency situation, requiring immediate admission for catheterization. The author is aware of an increased trend for GPs to catheterize such patients, when an urgent outpatient referral may be sufficient, provided the patient becomes pain free (see p. 77, 'Acute retention'). This may be a reflection of his practice, including some more remote parts of Scotland, but clearly this will avoid the patient having to make what must be a very uncomfortable journey to hospital.

Chronic retention

Chronic retention (see p. 79, 'Chronic retention') is not usually an emergency situation, unless it is complicated by renal failure – and indeed the symptoms of such may be why the patient consults. Chronic retention merits an urgent outpatient referral, but it is advisable to check the creatinine and electrolytes. If creatinine is >150, emergency admission is the safest course of action.

Severe or intractable symptoms

The improvement to be expected from current medical treatments is not usually dramatic, and unlikely to benefit a man with a high International Prostate Symptom Score (IPSS), particularly if his bothersome index is 5 or 6 (see Chapter 6). Patients in this category, or with moderately severe symptoms who fail to respond to medical treatment, require assessment by a urologist as surgery may be needed. When storage symptoms are predominant, especially if a flow rate measurement is not particularly low, they may indicate urodynamic assessment (and possibly cystoscopy – see below). With a history of retention, or episodes of prolonged delay before initiating micturition, surgery may be needed to avoid intractable retention.

Severe obstruction

Although urodynamic assessment is needed to confirm obstruction, a severe reduction of urine flow rate probably means that surgery is likely to be needed. Particularly if associated with a high residual urine, it also suggests a risk of developing retention.

Indications for referral for cystoscopy (see also Chapter 7)

There are some situations where a cystoscopy is indicated to exclude other pathology, when otherwise urological referral may be unnecessary. Local arrangements may exist for this to be done as a one-stop procedure.

Potential bladder cancer

Frank (visible) haematuria should only be ascribed to prostatic disease by a process of exclusion. Investigation to exclude a bladder (or renal) tumour is essential and appropriate urgent referral (through a fast-track or one-stop haematuria service if available) is essential. With occult ('dipstick') haematuria, the incidence of bladder cancer is much lower than with frank haematuria and in a man of this age group, alternative benign causes are more likely. In general, investigation is recommended although the urgency is probably less unless it is associated with a sudden onset of severe storage symptoms, which in themselves are an indication for cystoscopy.

Urethral stricture

This diagnosis should be remembered as an alternative cause of outflow obstruction, especially if the patient is younger than usual. If a flow rate tracing is available, there is often a characteristic flat topped shape to the curve (see Figure 7.1e). A history of perineal or pelvic trauma, urethritis,

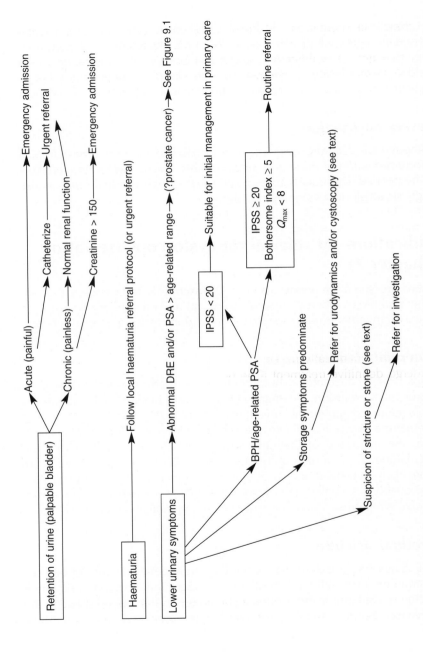

Figure 9.2 Suggested referral pathway for men with symptoms suggestive of prostatic disease.

urethral instrumentation or catheterization also raises this as a possible diagnosis. It is worth remembering that catherization is often performed during major surgical operations (including cardiac surgery), or following severe trauma, etc., but may not be volunteered by the patient.

Bladder calculi

These are less common than in the past and, as less imaging is now done for routine assessment of lower urinary symptoms, may be overlooked. Indeed, a calculus is sometimes first diagnosed when the patient's bladder is inspected at the time of a transurethral resection of the prostate (TURP). It may be a cause of storage symptoms, and should be suspected if there is a history of sudden stoppage of urine flow, or bladder or penile pain, especially if this is positional.

The patient as an individual

The guidance in this chapter does not override sensible clinical judgement. While it provides a basis for rational referral, each patient is an individual and indeed his own wishes and aspirations will determine what action is finally taken. For example, if, following informed discussion, a man with a minimally raised PSA indicates that he would not wish to undergo definitive treatment if he proved to have early prostate cancer, referral for invasive investigations (see Chapter 12) may not be appropriate. Similarly, while haematuria is normally an indication for urgent referral, this would clearly not be appropriate for a man bed-ridden with a terminal illness. Equally, as increasing numbers of men remain in excellent health into their 80s and 90s, the caveats on radical treatment in the 'elderly' may need relaxation. An inevitable and highly desirable consequence of increasing care in the community is that communication between the primary and secondary care will improve and local protocols develop. It is in such an atmosphere of mutual respect and co-operation that the needs of the man with prostatic disease can be best served.

'Patient choice'

For conditions, both BPH and cancer, when only a small proportion of patients will have an actual surgical operation, and for which there would seem to be such advantages in developing local management protocols between primary and secondary care, having a choice of where to be treated seems less advantageous than it might with conditions where treatment decisions are more straightforward. However, where a patient is wishing to exert his right to choose, the information on management in secondary care that follows will be helpful. If, for example, it is likely that a man, if he had cancer, would opt for a radical prostatectomy, this might influence a decision about where he should go. However, one should bear in mind that the unit with the best surgical outcome from radical prostatectomy may not necessarily be the best for other aspects of managing the disease. Also, a long journey for a single surgical episode is a different matter from regular cancer follow-up in a man of advancing years.

10 WHAT HAPPENS IN THE UROLOGY DEPARTMENT: BENIGN PROSTATE DISEASE

Management points

- Basic assessment will still require International Prostate Symptom Score (IPSS) and flow studies, PSA (where appropriate), unless results are available from GP, and digital rectal examination (DRE).
- Usually, there is no absolute indication for surgery; the decision is made after informed discussion with patient.
- It is usual to confirm bladder outflow obstruction (BOO) by urodynamics – filling and voiding cystometrograms – prior to final decision to operate. If poor stream is due to weak detrusor muscle – low pressure, low flow – surgery is unlikely to be of benefit.

Conventional surgery

- Most (>90%) of prostate operations are transurethal resections (TURPs).
- Open operations, usually retropubic prostatectomy (RPP), are reserved for very large glands or occasional complicated situations.
- NEITHER OPERATION REMOVES THE WHOLE PROSTATE GLAND.
- They do not prevent the possible development of prostate cancer in the future.
- Relapse of benign prostatic hyperplasia (BPH) can occur with a re-operation rate of up to 15% over 8 years after TURP and 4.5% after RPP.
- The main post-operative complication is haemorrhage, followed by extravasation of urine.
- Mortality is low.
- The commonest long-term complication is retrograde ejaculation (>70%) about which warning is mandatory; erectile failure occurs but is less common (<15%).

- Urinary incontinence occurs in <1%.
- Urethral or bladder neck stricture requires operation in about 5% and should be considered if voiding symptoms recur.

Post-operative care
- Discharge from hospital is usual within 48 hours of TURP.
- Heavy lifting, sexual intercourse and driving should be avoided, building up to normal activity over 4–6 weeks.
- Passage of debris and small amounts of blood occur over the first few weeks.
- Major secondary haemorrhage may occur during second or third week, often associated with infection, but may need readmission and temporary catheterization.
- Epididymitis (3.0%) seems less common than in the past.

Alternative interventions
- These should still be considered investigative procedures and are not generally available.
- Thermotherapy has largely been abandoned.
- Laser techniques may become standard in future.
- Patients frequently seek alternative treatments as being 'better'.
- Standard surgical techniques have been perfected and outcomes understood.
- TURP can be considered as the archetypal 'minimally invasive' operation.

The urologist's role

Unless already available, the initial assessment described in Chapters 7 and 8 are essential. Most urology departments will have a nurse-led clinic in which these will be performed prior to consultation with the urologist.

While medical treatment is often initiated in the urology clinic, the essential role of the urologist is to determine the need for and to initiate surgical treatment. There are few absolute indications for surgery. In most instances the likely advantages and the potential side effects should be discussed with the patient who will make the final decision. Advice from the urologist will take into account the severity of the patient's symptoms and degree of obstruction. Although transurethral surgery has an admirable safety record, no surgical procedure is without hazard, and the patient's general condition must also be taken into account.

Indications for surgery

Will surgery be effective?

Despite the ageing population, the number of prostate operations for BPH is declining. This is in part due to improved pre-operative selection, but is mainly a reflection of the increasing use of medical treatment in those with mild-to-moderate symptoms. Surgery is principally indicated for those with severe symptoms associated with proven significant obstruction, and following an unsatisfactory response to medical treatment. Surgery is associated with a clear risk of side effects. Studies have shown that those most satisfied with the outcome of an operation are those with the most severe symptoms – otherwise, they might simply replace one set of symptoms with others equally troublesome.

Surgery is only likely to be successful if there is proven obstruction. In most instances, the patient should undergo urodynamic assessment (see p. 52, 'Urodynamics') before finally being offered surgery. A severely reduced flow rate can be due to an atonic detrusor muscle without actual obstruction. This is an intractable situation, but not one likely to be helped by surgery. Urodynamics are particularly important in those with severe storage symptoms, where inappropriate surgery might end in disastrous incontinence.

Complications of surgery

In making the final decision to undergo an operation, the patient must be aware of the possible consequences.

Whether a transurethral resection of the prostate (TURP) or open operation is performed, similar long-term problems may occur. In addition to removal of prostatic tissue, the operation inevitably destroys the bladder neck (internal sphincter). They will be relying on the external sphincter for continence. Rarely, as a result of trauma, or following surgical repair of a urethral stricture (urethroplasty), the external sphincter may have been compromised. This is perhaps the only absolute contraindication to surgery for BPH, as total incontinence would then be inevitable. Otherwise, the importance of preserving the external sphincter is central to the operative technique. Fortunately incontinence is rare, but it can occur.

Destruction of the bladder neck means that >70% of patients will experience retrograde ejaculation. Sexual function is otherwise not usually affected. However, men complaining of erectile failure often date its start to a prostate operation. This may be a non-specific effect in a man with waning potency and can occur after any operation. However, the cavernosal nerves essential for erection lie close to the prostate (see p. 6, 'Position and relationships') and perhaps they are compromised from time to time by minor extravasation of fluid or a periprostatic haematoma that was not otherwise apparent.

The main peri-operative complication is bleeding, which can occasionally be life threatening, but also causes clot retention. It is largely to clear any blood clots that the patient is catheterized post-operatively (catheterization is not essential after TURP but very few urologists omit this). The patient should be warned that mild or intermittent bleeding is likely for a few weeks, and if this happens, to increase his fluid intake. Significant secondary haemorrhage, commonest in the second or third post-operative week, which may be associated with infection, can be severe enough to require re-admission and catheterization.

Extravasation of urine can occur due to breach of the 'capsule' during transurethral resection, or from inadequate closure or breakdown of the suture line after open operation. After open operation, it is normal to insert a drain, which may leak urine for a day or two. Rarely, operative insertion of a drain may be necessary if serious extravasation occurs after TURP.

It is important to emphasize that this is not a 'prostatectomy' in the sense of complete removal of the prostate gland. As a result, recurrence of the obstruction due to regrowth of BPH tissue is possible with reported re-operation rates after 8 years ranging from 5 to 15.5% following TURP and from 1.8 to 4.5% after open operation. Neither operation prevents subsequent development of prostate cancer and, indeed, will not necessarily diagnose cancer confined to the peripheral zone (see p. 8, 'Structure of the prostate' and p. 22, 'Symptoms and consequences of prostate cancer').

Operations for benign enlargement

In the middle of the last century, *transurethral resection of the prostate* (TURP) replaced open surgery as the standard procedure. A small number of open operations (*retropubic or transvesical prostatectomy –* see p. 6, 'Position and relationships') are still performed, mainly to deal with the extremely large prostate for which a TURP would be impractical and risk undue blood loss. An open operation is sometimes appropriate in conjunction with another procedure, for example removal of a large calculus from the bladder. While usually the decision is made electively, in borderline cases, the patient may be asked to consent to either, and the decision made by the surgeon at a preliminary cystoscopy. Very rarely, excessive bleeding during a TURP may necessitate conversion to an open operation. Both open operation and TURP aim to remove the benignly enlarged tissue as completely as possible, leaving the surgical 'capsule' – the attenuated peripheral zone (see p. 13, 'Pathology of benign prostatic enlargement'). This is more readily achieved by an open operation. On the other hand, manually extracting the benign tissue in a small prostate is difficult as the plane of enucleation is less well developed.

Bladder neck incision (BNI)/transurethral incision of prostate (TUIP)

These terms describe the same procedure, TUIP being the term used in the USA and increasingly in the UK. Mainly appropriate for the small prostate, using a point rather than a loop on the resectoscope, one or two cuts are made across the bladder neck and down the length of the prostate. From the patient's point of view, the operation is similar to a TURP, although there is usually less bleeding. A similar operation is used for treating bladder neck stenosis which can complicate a TURP, and for bladder neck hypertrophy (see p. 18, 'Differential diagnosis') in younger men. The re-operation rate probably is higher than after TURP, but the reported data for TUIP shows wide variations in incidence.

Post-operative care

The catheter is usually removed within 48 hours (perhaps a day or two longer after open surgery). Occasionally, patients find it difficult to pass urine and need recatheterization at this stage. If voiding is still difficult, he may be sent home with a catheter for a few weeks. Usually, when this catheter is removed, all is well, but very rarely the problem might be due to a small piece of residual tissue which will require re-resection. Problems voiding are more likely to occur in a man with low-pressure chronic retention, or if there is an atonic bladder – hence the importance of pre-operative urodynamics. It can also occur after retention following pelvic surgery (particularly abdominoperineal resection of the rectum), when there may be bladder denervation.

Initially, frequency and other storage symptoms may continue or even deteriorate. The absence of an incision will encourage the patient to expect rapid recovery. He should be counselled that TURP, despite this, is a fairly major procedure, which leaves a raw area, which can be likened to a deep burn, over the surface of the prostate. Healing will take at least 6 weeks, and full recovery, both generally, and with regard to local symptoms, will require this period of time. Although post-operative urinary infections are common, they will usually be associated with dysuria.

New technologies in the treatment of BPH

A variety of alternatives to surgery have been developed. Some have come and gone, some may be destined to stay, and might ultimately replace the current operations. *Transurethral vapourization* is closest to conventional TURP, where the prostatic tissue is destroyed using a special attachment, rather than cut away. Destruction of the prostate by heating it (*thermotherapy* and *hyperthermia*) has probably passed into oblivion. Procedures using lasers are more promising. A laser beam can be used to incise the prostate, or more effectively to enucleate the enlarged tissue, which is then morcellated (i.e. mashed up) with a special device. This is more a minimally invasive version of an open operation than a TURP. *Green light laser* is a device for destroying prostatic tissue. The latter has received a lot of publicity, as indeed have a number of these developments. This in turn creates a demand from patients. Currently, their availability is limited by the small number of centres which have the (often expensive) equipment. This is as it should be, since until experience has confirmed their safety and efficacy, it would be unwise for them to be introduced generally. Whatever their apparent advantages, this should be emphasized to patients, and it can be pointed out that TURP is as much a minimally invasive procedure as is laparoscopy, and indeed could be considered as the original 'keyhole' surgical operation.

11   RETENTION OF URINE

Management points

Acute retention

- Is treated by catheterization.
- This can be done in primary care; if so, emergency admission may not be necessary.
- A trial without catheter is normally appropriate.
- Precipitating factors, such as constipation, should be first corrected.
- Success is increased if an α-blocker is prescribed.
- If pain persists after catheterization, it may not be due to the retention and the patient should be admitted.

Chronic retention

- If painless and with normal renal function does not require immediate catheterization.
- Urgent referral is recommended.
- When complicated by renal failure, this normally resolves on catheterization – hospital admission is advised as IV fluids may be needed, and occasionally dialysis.

Acute retention

Although it might be hoped that earlier treatment could prevent this complication, it remains a common emergency. It may be that men at risk have voiding symptoms that are less bothersome than frequency, etc. Certainly, men who develop retention often have never consulted about lower urinary tract symptoms (LUTS), and in the days of long waiting lists, very few men developed retention while waiting for prostatic surgery. A number of men admitted in retention are constipated and clearing the bowel allows spontaneous micturition. When there is an identifiable cause, it is essential that this is resolved before the catheter is removed, otherwise re-retention will occur.

Conventionally, men with retention are admitted and catheterized, then wait for the next available operating slot for an operation. However, things can be managed differently.

- When the skills are available, catheterization in primary care is perfectly reasonable, alleviates the man's pain sooner and spares him an uncomfortable journey. If he is catheterized, and catheter care at home is possible, there is no need for emergency admission, although checking his serum creatinine is probably worthwhile (see below). An urgent outpatient appointment is appropriate, unless the local urologist is prepared to organize a direct admission.
- Although, if admitted for catheterization, it is usual to keep him in hospital, a few departments may send him home and arrange for later admission.
- In most circumstances, after any precipitating causes (notably constipation) have been corrected, a trial without the catheter is worthwhile. There is good evidence that prescribing an α-blocker (see p. 58, 'Medical treatment of BPH') will increase the success rate, and this is now routine practice in most departments. A trial of catheter removal is less likely to be successful if there is pre-existing chronic retention (residual urine >1 litre), and probably not worthwhile if more than 2 litres is drained. If successful, the patient can be assessed as an outpatient and may be recommended to have an elective transurethral resection of the prostate (TURP) if indicated.
- It is well recognized that elective surgery has fewer complications than an operation performed immediately after an episode of retention.

Three words of warning

- The pain of acute retention is relieved instantly the catheter is passed. If pain persists, it may be due to an acute abdominal condition either precipitating retention, or drawing attention to coincidental chronic retention. If after catheterization in primary care the patient remains in pain, he should be admitted as an emergency.
- Acute retention and catheterization can cause a 'spurious' rise in PSA. The PSA should be measured in a man with retention when the prostate is clinically malignant – this is to rule out a very high PSA, when early treatment for metastatic disease might be needed.

Otherwise, there will be less confusion and unnecessary worry if measurement is delayed (then performed according to the guidance on p. 33, 'PSA as a diagnostic or screening test').

- Acute retention can be a presentation of neurological disease, especially central disc prolapse and spinal metastases. Be conscious of a history of back pain, or of lower limb sensory or motor symptoms.

Chronic retention

Unless associated with severe symptoms, or renal failure, chronic retention is not an indication for immediate catheterization. The patient should be referred urgently and early surgery will probably be advised. However, there are some, usually elderly, men who seem to be relatively asymptomatic and don't come to any harm from their retention, and if their age and health contraindicate surgery, may well best be left alone. Unfortunately, men with long-standing chronic retention often find it difficult to pass urine after surgery, and even if they do, will often not be able to empty their bladders completely.

Unless long-standing, renal failure due to chronic retention usually resolves rapidly after catheterization. This is usually associated with a diuresis. Although this is partly the correction of fluid retention, it is usual to cover the initial recovery period with an intravenous infusion.

A note about catheterization

The old practice of slowly 'decompressing' the bladder has no proven value. It is true that occasionally, following relief of retention, bleeding will occur from the bladder. However, this will occur however fast the urine is drained. Similarly, intermittently clamping the catheter 'to maintain bladder tone' is unnecessary.

12 PROSTATE CANCER: PRESENTATION AND ASSESSMENT IN PRIMARY CARE

Management points

Presentation

- Lower urinary symptoms. These may be due to the cancer itself, but usually only when locally advanced, or they may be due to benign prostatic hyperplasia (BPH), with the cancer diagnosed coincidentally during investigation.
- Locally advanced disease may be diagnosed on digital rectal examination (DRE) done for any reason, or may present with outflow symptoms, retention or invasion of the ureters causing obstructive renal failure. Rectal symptoms, or lower limb oedema due to vascular or lymphatic obstruction, are rare presentations.
- Metastatic disease usually presents as bone pain, but pathological fracture or spinal cord compression may be first manifestation of the disease. General debilitation, or non-skeletal metastases are unusual in the absence of bony metastases.
- Asymptomatic disease is increasingly diagnosed as a result of PSA testing (see Chapter 5).

Diagnosis

- In primary care, clinical examination and PSA estimation are the main factors in alerting to the need for referral.
- The use and limitations of PSA testing are covered in full in Chapter 5.
- In dealing with a request from a patient to have a PSA test, appropriate counselling is mandatory.
- Although not strictly in accord with current guidelines, the author would recommend a DRE at such time, to avoid a man with

asymptomatic, but clinically overt, cancer declining to proceed with PSA testing.

- Otherwise, DRE is not a sensitive method of picking up early prostate carcinoma.
- PSA is appropriate for the investigation of back pain or other symptoms suspicious of metastatic cancer.
- In excluding metastases, a PSA <10 is strongly reassuring; with metastases PSA >20 or indeed much higher, is usual.
- Immediate further investigation of PSA at this level is only necessary for those in whom radical treatment of early cancer is appropriate (see below), although a period of monitoring may be wise in some cases.

Referral (see also Chapter 9)

- Urgency of referral with possible early prostate cancer (no evidence of disease on DRE, PSA <20) is now governed more by NHS targets than biological necessity.
- Unlike most cancers, there is little evidence that treatment within 2 months will have any effect on outcome.
- The need for radical treatment to be commenced within 2 months will dictate referral patterns for those in whom radical (curative) treatment would be considered.
- Where radical treatment would not be appropriate, a more relaxed referral is possible without detriment to the patient. Local protocols may exist and should be followed.
- Local practice will vary. Some urology units will use their Prostate Assessment Clinic for prostate cancer referrals; others will have separate 'fast-track' protocols.
- Urgent referral. Most guidelines advise urgent referral if PSA >20. This is because metastatic disease is then a possibility. Although uncommon, it is essential to pre-empt catastrophic complications of metastatic disease such as spinal cord compression.
- If he has a very high PSA (>100) and back pain, a telephone consultation is wise – immediate hormone treatment prior to hospital consultation might be advised.
- With signs or symptoms suspicious of actual or impending spinal cord compression emergency admission is mandatory as prompt treatment may prevent permanent disability. This applies equally to men known to have prostate cancer.

Among soft tissue cancers, carcinoma of the prostate presents some unusual features which bear uniquely on its management. Prostate cancer is now among the commonest of malignancies in the male, with over 20 000 cases diagnosed in the UK per year. Occult carcinoma occurs in 30% of those aged over 50 (p. 20, 'Pathology and epidemiology of prostate cancer') but most will go to their graves without knowledge of this disease lurking in their prostates. Prostatic adenocarcinoma is perhaps unique among cancers in that for many who are diagnosed with the disease, treatment (with potential for harm) is not needed immediately and indeed may never be needed. Treatment for prostatic metastases is far more effective than that available for most other forms of metastatic cancer. The paradoxes created by this disease exercise urologists, oncologists and scientists in equal measure. Its diagnosis in a man for whom cure is necessary will be of immeasurable benefit. Where he is not so at risk, it will merely be a cause of anxiety. Justifiable PSA testing to exclude possible metastatic disease will bring to light cases of localized disease; whether these require pursuit requires judgement and tact. For this particular disease recently introduced cancer treatment targets probably are inappropriate and may be counterproductive.

Presentation – see also p. 22, 'Symptoms and consequences of prostate cancer'

Prostate cancer will often present with lower urinary symptoms; it will certainly be the principal concern of many men who report such symptoms to their GP. As indicated on p. 20, 'Pathology and epidemiology of prostate cancer', most cancers develop in the peripheral zone and symptoms actually due to prostate cancer usually occur only late in the disease. Cancer often occurs in those without symptoms, and some would question whether measuring PSA in men with lower urinary tract symptoms (LUTS) is anything more than opportunist 'screening'. A digital rectal examination (DRE) is worthwhile, as men still do present with a hard craggy prostate but 'normal' or 'benign' findings on DRE do not exclude a carcinoma. Sometimes an advanced cancer, not causing symptoms of concern to the patient, will be picked up coincidently on a DRE done for another reason.

Locally advanced disease may present with retention of urine or renal failure due to ureteric obstruction. Invasion of the root of the penis may rarely cause priapism or erectile dysfunction but prostate cancer is not an issue for the vast majority of men who complain of this, and most urologists would not recommend PSA as a routine test in assessing erectile dysfunction.

Metastatic disease normally presents with bone pain. Musculoskeletal pain is common in the 'prostate cancer' age group but prostate cancer is a diagnosis to be remembered in a man whose pain is of recent origin or is atypical. Occasionally, pathological fracture or symptoms of impending or actual spinal cord compression may be its first manifestation. Fortunately, PSA is very helpful here, as most men with a significant metastatic load will have very high levels, often in excess of a thousand. Similarly, a PSA of <10 will confidently rule out metastatic disease in almost all cases. Note that early prostate cancer and benign backache are both common and frequently coexist. Unless the patient would be a candidate for curative treatment of early disease (see below), a PSA, measured to exclude metastatic disease, of less than 10 should be treated as a 'negative' result. The principal difficulty arises when PSA is in the range 10–50, where metastatic disease is possible but unlikely. Here a telephone consultation with a urologist is worthwhile, and for further investigation, a bone scan might be the best option, rather than an invasive prostatic biopsy.

Other sites of metastases are unusual (see p. 22, 'Symptoms and consequences of prostate cancer'), except in terminal disease, and rare in the absence of bone metastases as well. PSA levels in 'carcinomatosis' due to prostate cancer are likely to very high.

These are the classic presentations of prostate cancer, but in 2007, the most common entry into a diagnostic pathway is following a PSA test, done for whatever reason, and increasingly at the request of the patient himself. The issues addressed in Chapter 5 are not reconsidered here, but in deciding how to proceed in the face of a 'raised' PSA, or request for it to be measured, each patient, his health, age and aspirations, must be considered.

Diagnosis of prostate cancer

In all but a few instances, the diagnosis and treatment of prostate cancer can only be commenced following a histological diagnosis. This normally is obtained by a biopsy of the prostate, usually performed with the aid of transrectal ultrasound, but on occasion the diagnosis may come from a lymph node or bone biopsy. Although no longer the principal method of obtaining tissue, some cases of prostate cancer will still come to light following a transurethral resection of the prostate (TURP) done for presumed benign disease. Clearly these are within the province of the hospital service; the role of the general practitioner is to identify those in whom the disease is likely and to make the appropriate referral.

Referral

The algorithm in Chapter 9 (Figure 9.1, p. 65) is a guide to the referral for a man with a raised PSA. Disease curable by radical local treatment, be it surgery or radiotherapy, has a good prognosis for survival, and a slow progression rate. Thus delays in treatment, even of many months, will not affect the outcome. It is only when the patient has advanced, symptomatic, or life-threatening disease that there is the urgency usual for other types of cancer. However, the management of prostate cancer is now covered by the NHS targets for cancer treatment, demanding that treatment is commenced within 2 months of referral. This provides a considerable challenge when dealing with the man with a raised PSA, since the majority will not have cancer, and many who do will not come to surgical or other radical treatments. How this is dealt with is a matter for local decision, and is outside the scope of this book. However, the basis for urgent referral should be:

- Has he severe symptoms?
- Is there a possibility of imminent dangerous progression?
- If he has asymptomatic disease, is he a candidate for radical treatment?

Allaying anxiety is also important, and this does justify an early appointment. On the other hand, the fact that a referral is considered urgent might paradoxically increase rather the reduce anxiety.

When is urgent referral mandatory?

Urgent attention is needed if the patient has pain from metastases, or is in imminent danger of developing a serious complication such as spinal cord compression or renal failure. Most guidelines suggest urgent referral of all men with PSA >20. At this level, the possibility of a benign cause is small, and there is the possibility that the patient may have metastases or sufficiently advanced local disease to risk complications.

When the patient has symptoms of metastatic disease such as back pain, and a substantially raised PSA (>100) a telephone consultation prior to referral is wise. This is one circumstance in which treatment without prior histological confirmation may be appropriate, and in severe cases the urologist or oncologist may recommend treatment be started before he or she sees the patient.

The most critical issue is spinal cord compression. If this is dealt with in time, disability can be prevented, but once paralysis is established, irreversible damage will have occurred. In a man already being treated for prostate cancer, prompt spinal decompression or radiotherapy may well still be effective in preventing permanent paralysis. Actual or impending spinal cord compression is an indication for emergency admission.

13 PROSTATE CANCER: INVESTIGATION

Management points

Diagnostic tests (mainly appropriate in secondary care)

- Histological confirmation is essential in most cases. Usually, the prostate is biopsied per rectum under guidance of transrectal ultrasound (TRUS).
- The complications of this procedure are bleeding, septicaemia and a significant incidence of false negative results.
- A negative biopsy does not exclude cancer – follow-up with monitoring of PSA, and often further biopsies, are needed.
- Imaging of the prostate has little diagnostic significance. TRUS is principally used to ensure adequate sampling of the prostate. Imaging is used to stage the disease and plan treatment.
- Neither TRUS nor magnetic resonance (MR) imaging is fully reliable in assessing extracapsular spread.
- MR and CT scanning are also used to identify enlarged pelvic lymph nodes. A negative result does not exclude lymph node metastases.
- In imaging for metastatic disease, bone scintigraphy is the standard investigation, with a sensitivity far in excess of bone radiology. MR is more sensitive, is useful in distinguishing 'hot spots' from other causes, and is the investigation of choice to identify spinal cord compression.
- Ultrasound of the kidneys will identify obstruction in cases of ureteric involvement.

Biopsy

While in the past many, if not most, cases of prostate cancer were diagnosed from transurethral resection of the prostate (TURP) chips, in the current era of PSA testing, diagnosis is usually by a needle biopsy, performed per rectum with the assistance of transrectal ultrasound (TRUS) imaging. Although TRUS may identify abnormal areas from which to take extra biopsies, its main role is to ensure correct sampling of the gland. In advising a patient about this procedure, the following should be emphasized.

- *Discomfort and analgesia.* Normally, biopsy is done without general anaesthetic. Nowadays some form of local anaesthesia or analgesia usually is used, rather than relying on the stoicism of the patient. Techniques vary and it is worth consulting about local practice before advising patients.
- *Multiple* biopsies. In the past, six (sextant biopsy) were normal, but now eight, ten or more are more likely. The greater the number of biopsies, the greater is the chance of picking up the cancer (see below). A few urologists, in exceptional cases, will take as many as 20 biopsies but this usually requires a general anaesthetic.
- *Complications*
  Infection and septicaemia. Passing a needle into the prostate via the bacteria-laden rectum is clearly potentially hazardous. Optimal antibiotic regimens have been established to reduce this risk, but urinary infection and symptoms of septicaemia still occur from time to time. *Bleeding.* Haematomas in the prostate are common. Transient haematuria or slight rectal bleeding is unlikely to cause problems, but clearly the patient should be warned of the possibility. More severe bleeding can occur, particularly from (possibly aberrant) vessels in the wall of the rectum.
  The risk from these complications is not negligible and death from septicaemia has been reported.
- *Reliability.* As the biopsy technique can only sample the prostate, there is a significant chance of missing a tumour. With the sextant (six specimen) technique used in the past, a false-negative rate of 20% was reported with a substantial number of cancers diagnosed on repeat biopsy. Biopsy protocols now take more cores and target those parts of the gland most likely to harbour cancer. However, it remains difficult to completely exclude cancer on biopsy. As discussed in Chapter 5, this is a significant factor to be brought to the attention of a man seeking a PSA test – some 60% of those with a mildly 'raised' PSA will not have cancer, but for many it will be a long time, during which multiple biopsy sessions may be needed, before this can be confirmed.

Tumour grade

Biopsy establishes the diagnosis and grade of the tumour. The Gleason grading system, used almost universally, is an important guide to prognosis. Because of the variable patterns within prostate tumours, the two commonest are graded from 1 to 5, and then added to give a score of 2–10. Tumours with a score of 8–10 have a poor prognosis and in some situations might merit more aggressive treatment.

Tumour stage

Management, choice of treatment and prognosis, as with all forms of cancer, depend on the tumour stage. The International Union Against Cancer (UICC) TNM system is now almost universal (see Appendix 2). In practice, these define three clinical situations:

- *Confined disease.* If the tumour is contained within the capsule of the prostate (T1 and T2), and can be completely removed by surgery, it should be curable. Such tumours will have a good prognosis for other treatment modalities. Within this category, stage pT1c, tumour within a clinically benign gland detected by biopsy after PSA testing, is increasingly common. Traditionally pT1a and pT1b were identified from TURP chips on the basis of the percentage of tumour; if this is small (pT1a), the prognosis without treatment approaches normal life expectancy. Similarly, prognosis on needle biopsy relates to the amount of tumour (the number of involved needle cores or the proportion of tumour in each core).
- *Locally advanced disease.* When the tumour has extended through the capsule, cure becomes less likely. This stage varies from microscopic extension to clinically obvious local invasion, T3 or T4 disease, which might cause bladder outflow or ureteric obstruction. Locally advanced disease is still amenable to local treatments, but often more for palliation and control rather than in expectation of cure.
- *Metastatic disease*
  Lymph node metastases within the pelvis are difficult to diagnose. Their likelihood can be inferred from a combination of the tumour grade and extent of primary disease. They become important if curative surgery is planned, when a preliminary lymphadenectomy might first be performed. Conventionally, surgery would be

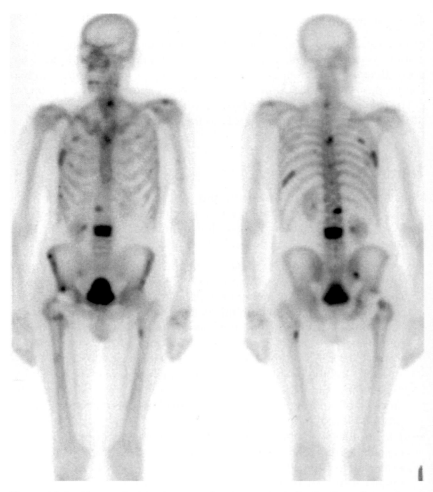

Figure 13.1 Bone scintigraphy scan showing typical distribution of prostate cancer metastases.

abandoned if frozen section revealed metastases in the nodes, although some surgeons will proceed if the metastases are small and/or few in number.

Distant metastases usually involve the axial skeleton. M1 disease is considered incurable by current methods, but is usually responsive to hormonal treatment.

Staging investigations

Images of the primary tumour can be obtained by TRUS, by MR imaging or from CT scans; most reliance is probably placed on MR. The aim is to detect capsular invasion, and no technique can do this accurately; both false-positive and false-negative results are common. Often the finger of an experienced urologist is as good at distinguishing between confined disease and local extension.

MR and CT may detect enlarged lymph nodes, but early metastases will occur in normal-sized nodes and nodal enlargement is not necessarily due to cancer. The extent to which these investigations are used varies. They are only appropriate where the result will influence treatment, and if so, lymph node biopsy may be needed.

The standard test for identifying metastatic disease is scintigraphy (bone scan – Figure 13.1), more sensitive than radiology, but non-specific. Benign bone or joint lesions will produce 'hotspots' on bone scans. Bone radiology is used to *exclude* other, non-malignant lesions. A hot spot with a normal x-ray is likely to be due to a metastasis. MR imaging is more accurate, useful in equivocal situations and an essential tool where spinal cord compression is suspected. Occasionally, a bone biopsy is the only way to distinguish metastatic disease from other conditions of the bone.

Other investigations

Ultrasound examination of the kidneys may be appropriate in advanced disease to exclude hydronephrosis.

In advanced disease, a full haematology and biochemistry screen is necessary. Bone alkaline phosphatase is a useful adjunct to PSA in monitoring response and progression of metastatic disease.

14 PROSTATE CANCER: TREATMENT OPTIONS

Management points

- The unusual nature of prostate cancer makes deferred treatment (active surveillance) an option for selected patients at most stages of the disease.
- Hormonal treatment as primary management, or neoadjuvant or adjuvant treatment may have a role throughout the disease spectrum.
- The standard hormone treatment is one of the luteinizing hormone releasing hormone (LHRH) analogues, currently available in monthly or 3-monthly depot preparations. As there is a risk of initial tumour flare, it is wise to cover the initial 3 weeks of treatment by prescribing an antiandrogen in addition.
- Subcapsular orchiectomy is therapeutically similar, and still preferred by some men.
- The principal side effects, loss of libido, hot flushes, lack of drive and loss of cognitive function, are similar for both, as are the long-term toxicities, loss of muscle mass, anaemia and reduced bone density with a risk of osteoporotic fractures.
- The antiandrogen bicalutamide (Casodex), licensed for treatment of locally advanced disease, may have fewer side effects. Cyproterone acetate (a progestogen) is no longer in long-term use because of liver toxicity; monitoring liver function of patients on bicalutamide is probably also wise.
- Other drugs, e.g. oestrogens, are rarely used.
- Combined treatment with LHRH analogue (or orchiectomy) and an antiandrogen is little used in the UK.
- Radical prostatectomy can cure confined disease. Its principal side effects are incontinence and erectile failure.
- External beam radiotherapy can cause rectal and bladder symptoms; toxicity and efficacy have been improved by newer techniques, conformal radiotherapy and intensity-modulated radiotherapy (IMRT).

- Brachytherapy, implanting radioactive seeds in the prostate, under transurethral ultrasound (TRUS) guidance is suitable for selected patients only.

Deferred treatment (active surveillance)

Prostate cancer is unusual; for many men treatment is not appropriate at diagnosis.

Deferred treatment in early disease

'Curative' treatment for prostate cancer is only possible in the early stages of the disease, when it is not immediately life threatening, and usually asymptomatic. It progresses slowly, with a prognosis for survival of many years, such that assessing efficacy of treatment requires 10 or 15 years' survival data. It is rare under the age of 50 and commonest in the elderly. With the increased use of PSA tests, more and more men with early prostate cancer are being diagnosed. It is inconceivable that treatment of *some* men with early disease will not prevent them dying from prostate cancer, but for many, radical treatment, which has a significant side-effect profile, will have no benefit, as their disease will not progress to produce symptoms or cancer death within their lifespan. It would be a major breakthrough in management if we had some way of accurately predicting those whose disease is life threatening and for whom aggressive treatment is necessary. Currently, this can be achieved by delaying treatment until there is evidence of progression. This is now termed 'active surveillance' (rather than 'watchful waiting'), which better describes what is being done – the patient is not being abandoned to his fate, but kept under close review for the first signs of tumour progression, when prompt treatment will be started.

Deferred treatment in advanced disease

In advanced disease, the argument is somewhat different. It has to be accepted then that the disease is incurable, and while treatments are effective, they have only a temporary benefit, with significant side effects. Whether they are more effective when started early rather than late remains a controversial subject and even if early treatment prolongs survival, this may be mitigated by the loss of quality of life from treatment-related side effects and toxicity. Here too, it can be argued that active surveillance and prompt treatment when symptoms or other manifestations of progression occur may be in the patient's best interest.

Deferred treatment: implications

At whatever stage of the disease, deferring treatment is far from being the easiest management option. Since it is often the more elderly man with limited life expectation for whom active surveillance is appropriate, it is easy to be accused of 'ageism' and it must be made clear to the patient that he is not being abandoned, or being denied treatment. The patient must be willing and able to be kept under close follow-up. This is probably not an option for a man living in a remote Scottish Highland croft. Most importantly, the general practitioner plays a vital role in promptly informing the urologist or oncologist of any change in the patient's condition that might herald progression of his disease.

Hormone treatment

The dependence of the prostate, and of most prostatic cancers, on testosterone (Figure 14.1) was the basis of *androgen deprivation* becoming one of the earliest effective systemic cancer treatments. Although we have come a long way from the days when every man even with a suspicion of the disease was started on large doses of oestrogens, hormone treatment still plays a part in managing all stages of the disease, and is the ultimate treatment for progressing disease however managed initially. Unfortunately, despite its short-term efficacy, the benefits are temporary and relapse is inevitable. The processes leading to *hormone refractory disease* are subject to much research. Understanding and overcoming hormone refractory disease would completely alter the outcome for men with prostate cancer. The benefits of hormone treatment have to be weighed against its significant side effects and toxicity.

Orchiectomy

This, the most direct method of androgen deprivation, was pretty well the standard treatment in the 1970s and 1980s. The stigma of 'castration' can be avoided by enucleation of the glandular tissue from the testes

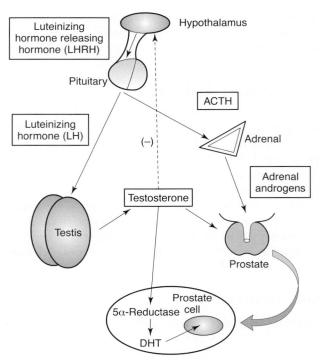

Figure 14.1 Hormonal regulation of prostate. Negative feedback from testis to hypothalamus regulates testosterone level. Note additional androgen drive from adrenal gland (controlled by adrenocorticotrophic hormone – ACTH). Conversion of testosterone to dihydrotestosterone (DHT) by 5α-reductase takes place in prostate cell cytoplasm.

(*subcapsular orchiectomy*), rather than their complete removal. It is still an option which appeals to a small number of men. Further compliance with treatment is not needed. It has an instantaneous effect and is the best choice in acute situations such as spinal cord compression.

LHRH analogues

These reduce testosterone levels to that equivalent to orchiectomy ('castrate range') by preventing the release of luteinizing hormone (LH) from the pituitary. A variety of sustained-release preparations are available with a frequency of injection ranging from 1 to 3 months (longer periods might become possible in future). Their therapeutic effects are identical – patients may need to be told that the longer-acting preparations containing more of the drug do not mean they are 'stronger'. The strategy for sustaining the release varies. Goserelin (Zoladex) is a pellet that is implanted subcutaneously, while others, e.g. leuprorelin (Prostap) and triptorelin (Decapeptyl), are suspensions given by sub-cutaneous or intramuscular injection. Differences such as the size of the needle and the period between injections (for some, strictly 12 weeks, others, 3 calendar months) may influence the choice in some patients.

Why 'agonist'? – tumour flare

These drugs are analogues of the natural LHRH peptide and were developed initially with a view to treating deficiency syndromes. Their immediate effect is indeed to stimulate LH release and hence testosterone secretion. However, after a few weeks, LH secretion is suppressed and testosterone levels fall to the castrate range. During the period of hyper-secretion, tumour growth may actually be stimulated. This might increase symptoms and cases of spinal cord compression from expansion of vertebral metastases have been reported. It is now standard practice to cover this period of 'flare' by administering an antiandrogen (see below), commencing a few days before the first LHRH agonist injection and continuing for at least 3 weeks after.

Side effects and toxicity

Other than the obvious differences in mode of delivery, and the initial flare from LHRH analogues, the side effects and toxicity of orchiectomy and LHRH analogues are essentially similar. Loss of libido and erectile failure, while not inevitable (18th century castratos were sexually active), are usual in men in the prostate cancer age group. Hot flushes, analogous to those experienced by post-menopausal women, occur in 25%. Most men tolerate these, but steroid replacement with a progestagen drug such as cyproterone acetate is helpful in troublesome cases. General reduction in physical drive is not unusual, and a loss of cognitive function has been reported. The latter is worth a warning if the patient is still working, or engaged in intellectual activity. In the long term, loss of muscle mass, anaemia and, most importantly, loss of bone density may occur. Osteoporotic fractures are the most significant long-term complication. Assessment of bone density should be considered after prolonged use.

Although orchiectomy and LHRH analogues do not cause the severe cardiovascular complications associated with oestrogen therapy (see below), the possibility of some residual toxicity is raised from time to time, and there is some experimental basis for this. There is evidence that diabetics may be most at risk. Although, as they are now the most commonly used method of androgen deprivation, these observations mainly relate to LHRH analogue treatment, there is no reason to suppose they do not equally apply to patients who have undergone orchiectomy.

Antiandrogens

An alternative to reducing serum levels of testosterone is to block its action with antiandrogens, of which there are two types. Steroidal drugs are progesterone agents, which have an additional central effect similar to oestrogens (see below). *Cyproterone acetate* was a useful alternative to orchiectomy before LHRH analogues became available. However, it causes a significant incidence of potentially fatal liver damage precluding its use in long-term treatment. It is still commonly prescribed to prevent tumour flare when starting LHRH analogue treatment.

There are a number of purely antagonistic *non-steroidal antiandrogens*, which do not inhibit testosterone secretion. For practical purposes, the only drug now in use is *bicalutamide (Casodex)*. Its licensed role has been sharply defined by clinical trial results for use as monotherapy in advanced localized disease, or (in a lower dose) in combination with orchiectomy or LHRH analogue treatment (*combined androgen blockade*). These drugs can also cause liver damage, and monitoring liver function is wise during their use. Casodex can cause breast discomfort or gynaecomastia in a small but significant number of men. It is less likely to cause sexual dysfunction, and this is perhaps its main advantage. It is likely that other side effects of androgen deprivation, loss of muscle mass and bone density, are less of a problem. Hot flushes can occur but are less frequent than with orchiectomy or LHRH analogue treatment.

Other hormonal treatments

Oestrogens, especially *(diethyl)stilboesterol*, once the mainstay of prostate cancer treatment, have fallen out of use mainly because of cardiovascular toxicity. The toxicity mainly results from liver metabolites; parenterally administered oestrogens seem to have less toxicity, which might be further

98

reduced by concomitant prescription of aspirin. Although interest in revisiting oestrogen therapy remains on the research agenda, they currently have little use in routine clinical practice. *Ketoconazole,* in higher doses than as a fungicide, suppresses androgen secretion by both testes and adrenals. However, it can also cause general adrenal failure. *Aminoglutethimide* suppresses adrenal androgen secretion, which is also one of the actions of *corticosteroids* such as *prednisolone,* although the latter is now most commonly used in combination with cytotoxic chemotherapy in relapsed disease. LHRH *antagonists* have been under protracted development – they produce immediate effect, avoiding the risk of tumour flare, and may prove to have other advantages. Surgical adrenalectomy and hypophysectomy are largely historical treatments.

Combined androgen blockade

Theoretically a more intense reduction of the effects of androgen on the tumour would be achieved by combining either orchiectomy or LHRH analogue treatment with an antiandrogen. After initial encouraging reports, there was intense clinical research into this concept, with a number of randomized trials and meta-analyses. Suffice to say that any benefit in terms of improved survival is small, and in the UK at least, combined androgen blockade is little used.

Radical prostatectomy (Figure 14.2)

Perhaps what more accurately should be called 'total' prostatectomy involves complete removal of the prostate, along with the seminal vesicles, and reconstruction by anastomosis of the bladder neck to the urethra. The usual risks of any surgical procedure can occur, but overall mortality from radical prostatectomy is well below 1%. However, this is partly the result of selection – for those at risk from surgery, other options are available, and a man with co-morbidity sufficient to reduce his life expectation would not be a candidate for the operation anyway. The major intra-operative hazard is bleeding from the veins in front of the prostatic apex, which can occasionally be catastrophic. There is a small risk of injury to the rectum. The following specific long-term complications may occur.

- *Incontinence* results from the proximity of the bladder sphincter mechanism to the prostate. In the hands of an experienced surgeon,

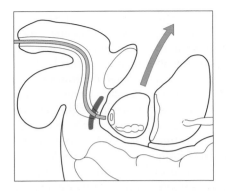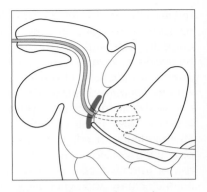

Figure 14.2 Radical prostatectomy. (Modified from Kirk D. *Understanding prostate disorders.* London: Family Doctor Publications Ltd in association with the British Medical Association, 2005)

the risk of severe incontinence should be small (<5%). A larger proportion may have occasional leakage on coughing or other stress, or simply have a feeling of insecurity sufficient to make them wear a small pad in their underpants. It is important to warn the patient that initial incontinence for a day or two after catheter removal is not unusual, but usually recovers. Patients are instructed in pelvic floor exercises to aid this process. Severe incontinence can be managed conservatively with external appliances or even a catheter. Many men feel this to be an adequate price to pay for elimination of their cancer. Full urinary control can be achieved by insertion of an artificial sphincter, but this does involve further complex surgery, with all the potential problems resulting from implantation of a mechanical device.

- *Stenosis* due to fibrosis of the narrow anastomosis between bladder and urethra occurs in up to 10% of cases, producing difficulty voiding or, paradoxically, overflow incontinence. Treatment is straightforward. Dilatation or endoscopic division of the stenosis will usually correct it permanently.
- *Erectile failure* was previously an almost universal complication of the operation. With improved understanding of the anatomy of the penile nerves it is now avoidable in many cases, provided preservation of the nerves does not compromise adequate removal of

100

the cancer. Reversible trauma to the nerves, or post-operative haematoma, increases the risk of erectile failure in the immediate post-operative period, and recovery is possible for as long as a year. Unless the nerves have been completely destroyed, treatment with phosphodiesterise 5 (PDE5) inhibitors such as sildenafil (Viagra) or other drugs is helpful, and indeed there is evidence that their routine use will speed recovery of spontaneous function. Under current UK regulations, prostate cancer and major pelvic surgery are both included in the list of conditions for which medical treatment for erectile failure is financed by the NHS. If oral treatment fails, other measures such as intracavernosal prostaglandin injections, or even insertion of an inflatable prosthesis, may be considered. Many men, adequately warned of this complication in advance, will accept it as a consequence of their treatment.

- *Other abnormalities of sexual function.* Removal of the prostate and seminal vesicles, and division of the vas deferens inevitably abolishes ejaculation (but not orgasm), and there is often an apparent shortening of the penis.

Open surgery

Open surgery is currently the most common method of radical prostatectomy. The retropubic approach, through a lower abdominal incision, is most frequently used, but a perineal approach has some advantages, with less discomfort and shorter recovery time. It is particularly indicated in an obese man. The urethro-vesical anastomosis is protected by a urethral catheter; as there is a risk of urinary leakage, a drainage tube is left in place, usually for 1–2 days. Rapid initial recovery is usual. Most men can go home within a few days, but usually are readmitted for a day or two after 2–3 weeks for removal of the catheter. Return to normal activity takes 6–8 weeks although, as with most abdominal operations, complete recovery may take several months.

Laparoscopic and robotic prostatectomy

In addition to the usual benefits of less post-operative pain and more rapid recovery, a laparoscopic prostatectomy has other advantages. There is improved visualization of the depths of the pelvis, and a continuous suturing technique is possible for the anastomosis, allowing the catheter to be removed in 3–4 days. The operation requires considerable experience both in conventional open prostatectomy and in laparoscopic surgery in general. A number of centres in Europe and the USA have large experience of the operation, which is being performed increasingly in the UK.

Robotic prostatectomy

The term 'robotic' prostatectomy is a misnomer, as the operation is essentially done by remote control, the surgeon sitting at a consul controlling a machine that manipulates the laparoscopic instruments. Manipulation is easier than with conventional laparoscopy, and the consul provides excellent three-dimensional vision for the operator. The cost of the equipment is formidable, but is being acquired in a number of centres in the UK.

It would be unrealistic to expect these new techniques, particularly robotic surgery, to become universally available in the near future. The conventional open operation is now a safe and well tolerated procedure, and longer-term follow-up is still needed to confirm that the new techniques are as effective in eradicating the cancer.

Which surgeon?

Radical prostatectomy is considered a testing operation, and there is no doubt that outcomes vary from surgeon to surgeon. Caseload is a major factor; NICE has laid down guidelines concerning minimum numbers of cases performed and audit of outcomes. Increasingly, major pelvic cancer surgery, including radical prostatectomy, will be concentrated in cancer centres doing more than 50 operations per year. This is one area in which patient choice might be appropriate. Enquiry as to numbers of operations a unit or a surgeon does per year, and individual outcome data on continence rates, etc., is probably appropriate. However, case mix and selection, as well as surgical expertise, may affect outcomes.

External beam radiotherapy

Radical radiotherapy regimens vary, but essentially involve daily treatments over a period of 4–6 weeks. Short-term systemic and local side effects are common. Inevitably, the radiation will affect the bladder and the rectum, causing storage (irritative) urinary symptoms and perhaps haematuria, and diarrhoea and rectal bleeding. Severe rectal symptoms can be helped by steroid suppositories or enemas.

The curative effect of radiotherapy is directly related to dose. This in turn is limited by the toxicity of the radiation to the normal tissues. Conformal radiotherapy shapes the radiation beam to that of the irradiated tissues, reducing the surrounding tissue damage, allowing a larger dose to be administered with less toxicity. Further improvement has come with intensity-modulated radiotherapy (IMRT) where the intensity of the beam can be increased over the tumour.

The ill effects will continue for some time after the treatment is finished, and it is realistic to warn the patient that the period of disability associated with radiotherapy is likely to match that for radical prostatectomy. Since swelling of the prostate can occur, the treatment might tip the man with bladder outflow obstruction (BOO) into retention, and indeed if this risk is high, he could be catheterized prior to starting treatment. Side effects can persist, albeit mildly in most cases. Continuing mild rectal bleeding, amounting to streaks of blood with the stools, is quite common. As the penile nerves come within the radiation field, erectile failure can also complicate radiotherapy, but in contrast to prostatectomy, the risk increases with time; in the long term there is perhaps little difference in the incidence of this side effect. Although radiation can affect the bladder sphincter, incontinence is less likely than after surgery. Occasional radiation-induced urethral strictures occur.

The most important long-term complication of radiotherapy is a second cancer, in this case usually of the recto-sigmoid. Since the presenting symptoms, change of bowel habit and bleeding, mimic the side effects of the radiotherapy itself, it is well to be aware of this possibility in the man whose symptoms persist or recur several years after treatment. Tissue destruction leading to prostato-rectal fistula formation is fortunately now rare due to improved radiotherapy techniques.

Currently, neoadjuvant hormonal treatment (see below) is usually given for 3 months (or longer) before commencing treatment. The radiotherapy regimen is initially planned with CT scans on a dummy machine ('simulator') both to calculate the dose and to position the beam using tattooed skin marks. Treatment will usually be given during daily out-patient visits. Where this is not possible for reasons of health or geography, most radiotherapy departments can provide some form of hotel-style accommodation.

As with surgeons, radiation oncologists vary in expertise, and increasingly specialize. While 'patient choice' is usually interpreted in the context of surgical operations, if the author were undergoing radiotherapy, he would wish it to be undertaken under the supervision of a specialist in treating the prostate with experience from managing a substantial caseload.

Brachytherapy

Interstitial radiotherapy, by implanting into the prostate radioactive seeds with a limited field of radiation, is an attractive concept for maximizing tumour dose and limiting toxicity. It found temporary favour in the 1970s when the seeds were implanted into the prostate at open surgery. With the development of transrectal ultrasound (TRUS), which enables accurate imaging of the prostate both for dose calculation and to guide placement of the seeds via needles passed through the perineum, there has been a resurgence of interest in the technique. For the patient there are considerable attractions in terms of time, convenience and, for most, low toxicity. This has created a demand which has been difficult to satisfy.

Although brachytherapy is sometimes used in combination with external beam radiotherapy for advanced tumours, as a monotherapy it is suitable only for a highly selected group of patients. These are men with small, clearly confined tumours, just those tumours that have the best prognosis, a factor that must contribute to the encouraging survival results. As a newer technique, modern ultrasound-guided brachytherapy has still a fairly short period of follow-up, so some caution is needed in assessing efficacy in a tumour where survival is measured over 10 or even 15 years. Brachytherapy is not possible following a TURP, or if the prostate is very large, unless it can be shrunk by preliminary hormone treatment. Although the proportion of men who experience side effects is small, intractable, severe lower urinary symptoms, which can be very difficult to treat, occur from time to time.

When the criteria for brachytherapy are satisfied, the treatment involves two sessions. At the first, the prostate is imaged, its size and anatomy assessed. Using this data, the dose, the number of seeds and their position is calculated, and at a second session, the seeds are implanted. The seeds – iodine-125 or palladium-103 – come in strands that are cut to the length that contains the required number of seeds to be inserted into each of the needles positioned in the prostate.

15 PROSTATE CANCER: TREATMENT OF CONFINED (T1/T2) DISEASE

Management points

- There is no clear evidence in favour of any one management strategy, radical prostatectomy, radiotherapy or active surveillance.
- Some data suggest improved survival after radical prostatectomy, which will be favoured for younger men.
- All the appropriate options should be discussed with the patient; the decision may be based more on the differences in potential side effects.
- Neoadjuvant hormone therapy is used before radiotherapy but not radical prostatectomy.
- Adjuvant treatment (hormonal or radiotherapy) may be used in those at high risk for recurrence. Routine use is still a matter for clinical trials.

Treatment options

Generally, early confined prostate cancer can be treated by surgery, i.e. radical prostatectomy, or by radiotherapy, either external beam treatment or brachytherapy. Active surveillance is also an option for many men. Comparison of outcomes from these treatments is difficult as each has their own, different, selection criteria. These criteria may also lead to different assessment. For example, men for whom radical prostatectomy is considered will be younger, fitter, and only have the operation if a preliminary biopsy of their pelvic lymph nodes is negative, while the lymph node status of a patient undergoing radiotherapy (who may on average be older and less fit) will not be known. Improvements in both surgery and radiotherapy techniques also invalidate comparisons with patients treated years ago.

Uncontrolled observational studies have suggested, particularly for high-grade tumours, that radical prostatectomy produces better average survival. A randomized Scandinavian study, initiated before PSA testing was common, and thus involving men with more advanced disease than now, demonstrated a small but significant survival benefit from surgery compared to active surveillance. However, this was at the expense of many men receiving unnecessary treatment (as they died from causes other than their prostate cancer). A large study in the UK (ProtecT), involving substantial populations in a number of centres, is comparing radical prostatectomy, radiotherapy and surveillance in men whose cancers have been identified from PSA screening.

Active surveillance

The rationale for no immediate treatment with active surveillance has been discussed. As the results of trials emerge, and with better methods of defining prognosis, the men for whom this is appropriate may be better identified. Although best recommended for the older man with better differentiated tumours (Gleason score <7), when presented with the issues, even quite young men may decide on this option – they perhaps have more to lose from the side effects of the standard treatments.

Deciding on treatment

Meanwhile, it is difficult to recommend a definite 'best' treatment. Each treatment has its own set of side effects and complications, and for many these will be more important than any possible difference in therapeutic benefit. Radical prostatectomy will be considered more for the younger, fitter man, and surveillance for the man with a short life expectation. However, it is essential that all the options are discussed in a balanced way with every patient. Many urology and oncology departments now employ counselling nurses to do this. The patient does require time to consider the options and there is no evidence that a delay of even a few months will adversely affect the outcome of whatever treatment is chosen. For this particular tumour, the perception that it is important to 'catch cancer in time' does not apply, and the current targets for cancer treatment times may not be appropriate. Indeed, it may actually be harmful if hastening treatment denies the patient due opportunity to consider what is in his best interests.

Other treatments

New technology is finding its way into the management of prostate cancer. Local destruction of the tumour using lasers or high-intensity focused ultrasound (HIFU) has been proposed. Review of radical prostatectomy specimens has shown that even when a clearly defined tumour has been recognized on imaging, the disease process is often diffuse or multifocal, which is likely to limit the benefits from this type of approach. Freezing the prostate (cryotherapy) is not a new idea but is undergoing resurgence with the technology now available to localize and regulate the freezing. If it comes to have a role, it may be more to deal with relapse after conventional treatment rather than primary management. With publicity in the media, many men seek these treatments. Clearly, they will only be available as investigative techniques in a few centres and patients should be cautioned on the wisdom of sticking with the standard treatments.

Neoadjuvant hormone treatment

Androgen deprivation is not only an effective treatment for prostate cancer, it also produces a substantial reduction in the size of the prostate. Thus, benefits have been proposed from a period of hormone therapy prior to definitive treatment of the primary tumour.

Prior to surgery

For men undergoing radical prostatectomy, hormone therapy might reduce the percentage of cases where there was undetected spread of tumour beyond the capsule (pT3) – *downstaging*. Indeed, it was even suggested that overt T3 tumours could be made operable by this technique. While it is certainly the case that these objectives can be achieved at the time of surgery, benefit in terms of lower progression rates on follow-up does not seem to be realized. The treatment also causes local reaction, which makes surgery more difficult.

Prior to radiotherapy

The situation prior to radiotherapy is different. Here the aim is to reduce the size of both the tumour and the prostate itself, limiting the target for the radiotherapy field. This is achieved, and has been shown in studies to produce long-term benefit. Thus, most men undergoing radiotherapy are now offered a 3-month or longer period of neoadjuvant hormone treatment. Hormone treatment can also be used prior to brachytherapy to reduce a large prostate to within the limit of size for the technique.

Adjuvant hormone treatment

Routine treatment

Can the benefits demonstrated for women with breast cancer from early use of hormone drugs be reproduced in men with prostate cancer – is there a urological tamoxifen? To be acceptable, such a treatment must not only be effective but have minimal side effects. The most promising agent in this respect is bicalutamide (Casodex) and its use as adjuvant treatment has been studied in a related series of very large trials, in patients with early disease managed by surgery, radiotherapy and by surveillance. It would be expected that hormone treatment will delay progression in those whose disease has not been cured by their primary treatment and this is indeed the case. Would they do any worse if hormone treatment were delayed until progression occurred since, in many cases, the primary treatment might have cured the disease? There is now some patchy survival evidence coming through. In one instance this was negative and led to a recent revision of the licence for bicalutamide, withdrawing approval for its use in confined (stage T1) disease, although it remains a treatment option for locally advanced disease. Otherwise, whether routine adjuvant treatment for confined disease is beneficial remains an open question. Some of the trial data has reached the public domain and patients may wish to discuss it – such discussion perhaps is best conducted with the specialist who should have access to the latest data.

Adjuvant treatment in high-risk cases

Some patients are at high risk of treatment failure: after radical prostatectomy if the tumour is found to extend beyond the surgical margin or the lymph nodes are involved, or when PSA remains detectable; after radiotherapy when there has been a sub-optimal fall in PSA; in all cases where the Gleason score is 8 or above. Should these patients be given immediate adjuvant treatment? On the other hand, some of them will be 'cured' by the local treatment. Although there is some persuasive evidence for early intervention, no trial has been done to show this to be definitely better than delaying treatment until there is clinical recurrence. Adjuvant treatment would usually be hormonal therapy, although positive margins after surgery may be treated with radiotherapy. Modern diagnosis, by detecting prostate cancer at an early stage, has led to this, a new category of 'advanced disease', for which the prognosis in terms of survival is still good and thus any treatment (and its side effects and cumulative toxicity) may have to continue for many years.

16   PROSTATE CANCER: MANAGEMENT OF ADVANCED DISEASE

Management points

- Locally advanced disease is usually incurable, but long survival with good disease control is possible.
- Radical prostatectomy is sometimes performed, but most patients are treated with radiotherapy.
- Neoadjuvant hormone treatment is indicated prior to radiotherapy.
- Adjuvant hormone treatment after radiotherapy improves survival.
- Metastatic disease is treated with hormone therapy on diagnosis.

Once disease has spread beyond the capsule of the prostate, curative treatment is less likely to be effective. Control of disease and prolongation of survival rather than cure become the main aims of management.

Locally advanced disease

In early T3 disease, radical prostatectomy is feasible, although nerve preservation is unlikely. Some men undoubtedly can be cured, but the main advantage is for local disease control. Early lymph node metastases do not, in the eyes of some urologists, necessarily preclude surgery. However, the mainstays of management of this phase of the disease are radiotherapy and hormone treatment, although surveillance still remains an option for some men.

Although hormone therapy is a systemic treatment, it is an extremely effective method of controlling the primary tumour. When prostate cancer presents with retention of urine, most men will be able to void urine without the need for surgery following a period of hormone treatment. It is in treating locally advanced disease that neoadjuvant hormone treatment prior to radiotherapy has the clearest benefit. There is also good evidence from clinical trials that survival after radiotherapy can be improved by giving 2–3 years of adjuvant hormone therapy. What is less clear is whether, in terms of survival, the radiotherapy adds anything to the benefits of hormone treatment alone: the subject of a current randomized trial. If hormone therapy alone is used, local tumour progression may be the first clinical manifestation of hormone refractory relapse; at that time, radiotherapy may be a useful palliative option (see p. 120, 'Hormone refractory disease').

Metastatic disease

Bone metastases may present with pain or, rarely, complications such as spinal cord compression or fracture, or be asymptomatic and detected when the patient is investigated. While deferring treatment until the metastases become painful is a possibility, the current consensus is that diagnosing metastatic disease is normally an indication for immediately commencing hormone treatment. In most cases, symptoms demanding treatment will occur within a short time and the risk of progression causing serious complications before treatment is started is real. When treatment is delayed there seems to be a continuing increased risk of, for example, spinal cord compression persisting even after treatment has been started. Flare prevention with an antiandrogen is essential at this stage of disease. The rapid response following orchiectomy makes this the method of choice for spinal cord compression, and also perhaps renal failure due to ureteric obstruction, although usually this will be treated initially by percutaneous nephrostomy or ureteric stents.

17 PROSTATE CANCER: FOLLOW-UP

Management points

- There is scope for sharing follow-up of men with prostate cancer between primary and secondary care.
- The mainstay of follow-up is PSA measurement.
- PSA rarely needs checking more than once in 3 months, except as confirmation when a change in level occurs.
- Care is needed if the primary care team and hospital department use different biochemistry laboratories.
- PSA is not entirely reliable and results must be considered in clinical context. Treat the patient not his PSA!
- Ensure in advance the patient is aware of the significance of PSA changes if and when they occur.
- After radical prostatectomy, PSA should be undetectable but occasionally a low but stable level of PSA can occur in the absence of residual cancer.
- Some PSA is usually detectable after radiotherapy – a rapid fall to a low level indicates a good prognosis.
- As long as the PSA response persists, other follow-up investigations are unnecessary – however, relapse after hormone therapy sometimes occurs without much increase in PSA.
- Monitoring alkaline phosphatase is useful in men with bone metastases.
- Prognosis depends on tumour stage and grade.
- Prognosis with well-differentiated confined tumours may approach natural life expectation. It is poorer with tumours of Gleason Score 8–10 but 5-year survival is still >50%.
- Locally advanced disease is not completely curable, but many men with slow-growing tumours may die from other diseases first.
- In metastatic disease, the response of PSA to treatment is a valuable prognostic guide – early relapse is likely if the fall in PSA is slow and remains high.

There is clear scope for co-operation between primary and secondary care in following up men with prostate cancer, and indeed in most instances the administration of luteinizing hormone replacement hormone (LHRH) analogue injections, or prescription of other drugs, will be delegated to the primary care team. Within urology and oncology departments, trained nurses are undertaking increasing amounts of follow-up; since the mainstay of follow-up is prostate specific antigen (PSA) measurements, this could readily take place in the local health centre.

PSA in follow-up

A few points about PSA monitoring need reiteration.

- PSA rarely needs measuring more than once in 3 months (and less frequently when disease is well stabilized), except for early repeat measurements to confirm an increase in PSA before changing treatment.
- The discrepancies between different methods of PSA assay must be remembered if a general practice uses a different laboratory from the hospital. Since long distance is a frequent reason for sharing care, this is not an uncommon situation.
- Changes in PSA must be considered in clinical context – a definite but slow increase might indicate a relapse, but one for which immediate action might not be needed. Conversely, after hormone treatment, relapse occasionally occurs without PSA increasing.
- It is all too easy to treat the PSA and not the patient. PSA is increasingly used as a surrogate for response and for progression. Biochemical relapse without recurrence detectable clinically or on imaging is common. A change in treatment might then produce a fall in PSA; whether this produces clinical benefit is often less clear.
- Patients can become fixated on their PSA level. While the result may be 'good news' when the disease has responded to treatment, they have to be prepared for the possibility of later 'bad news'. A clear explanation at the outset of the true significance of PSA and what changes mean – in particular that a small increase in PSA does not herald impending doom – may pre-empt unnecessary worry later. This is particularly important if the PSA is measured in primary care so the result is available at a hospital consultation. While simplifying

management, it can cause unnecessary worry if an adverse result is not put into the correct context.

The significance of actual PSA levels varies depending on the management selected.

After complete removal of the prostate, PSA should be undetectable, so a measurable PSA after *radical prostatectomy* usually indicates likely persistence, or recurrence, of disease. When the prostate remains, as with *radiotherapy or hormone treatment*, the PSA is likely to be detectable – here it is the rate of fall and the level reached that is important. A slow fall to a level above the 'normal' range heralds a poor prognosis. Under *active surveillance*, the PSA will inevitably increase. Here it is the rate of change that is important. A consistent rapid increase (doubling time <2 years) will prompt intervention.

Some caution is needed in interpreting apparent adverse measurements. Small amounts of benign prostatic hyperplasia (BPH) tissue can be left after an apparently adequate radical prostatectomy, producing a low but stable residual level of PSA. After radiotherapy, a delayed temporary rise and fall in PSA of no significance is frequently observed. Cancer progression usually produces a steady increase. A sudden sharp rise when the PSA has previously been stable should raise questions about the cause. When the patient still has a prostate, the alternative causes of PSA increase (infection, instrumentation, etc. – see Table 5.1) might still occur. It is always wise to repeat a PSA before acting, and often this will show a reassuring return to previous levels.

Because of its sensitivity in detecting relapse, other methods of follow-up are usually unnecessary until a change of PSA occurs. The only, occasional, exception is following hormone therapy, when relapse can occur either without a rise in PSA, or with one which is disproportionately small. In following up men with metastatic disease on hormone treatment, the risk of this occurring can be reduced by measuring, in addition, alkaline phosphatase as a marker of bone destruction.

Prognosis

'How long have I got?' is the cliché question from the newly diagnosed cancer patient. In most men with prostate cancer, it is possible to give an optimistic reply, but it is essential to be realistic as well.

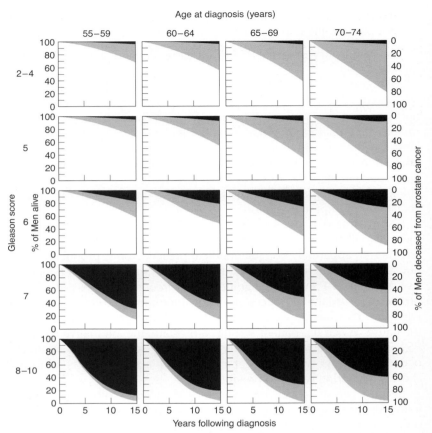

Figure 17.1 Mortality from prostate cancer related to age and tumour grade. Black areas represent percentage dying from prostate cancer, shaded from other diseases. (Reproduced with permission from Albertsen PC, Hanley JA, Gleason DF, Barry MJ. *Journal of the American Medical Association* 1998; **280**: 975–80)

Confined disease

The patient here is managed on the basis that the disease is either curable, or likely not to progress to a terminal stage within the patient's lifespan. The biology of the tumour probably has as much influence on the outcome as does how it is treated. Patients with well-differentiated disease have a prognosis approaching their normal life expectation. How much active treatment improves on this remains a moot point. Equally, patients with poorly differentiated disease (Gleason score 8–10) will have a much poorer prognosis (Figure 17.1). It is argued that so poor is the prognosis that inflicting the risks of surgery is not worthwhile. The alternative view, which the author holds, is that this group contains the very patients who have most to gain from surgery or other aggressive treatments. Even here, the 5-year survival is in excess of 50%.

Locally advanced disease

While eradication of the disease is unlikely when it has spread beyond the prostate, survival is still measured in years, and many men will still die from other causes. It is, however, much more likely that the disease will recur and that additional treatment will be needed. Here, it is important to be realistic, but to emphasize to the patient that further effective options are available should initial treatment fail.

Metastatic disease

Although most patients respond to hormonal treatment, it was always predicted that relapse would occur within 18 months and death within a further 6 months. The prognosis is now undoubtedly better, perhaps because PSA testing not only picks up 'curable' tumours, but also identifies advanced disease sooner than in the past. The response of PSA levels to hormone treatment is a valuable guide to prognosis. A slow fall of PSA to a level above the normal range is usually followed by an early relapse. A rapid fall to low levels (possibly below the lower limit of detection) is usually sustained for a long time, and when relapse does occur, there is a good chance of a response to second-line hormone treatment (see p. 120, 'Second-line hormone treatments).

18 PROSTATE CANCER: MANAGEMENT OF RELAPSED DISEASE

Management points

- A number of options are available in secondary care when curative treatment of early disease fails.
- Hormone refractory relapse represents the final phase of the disease, before terminal illness.
- Second-line hormonal treatment is useful after good response to primary hormone treatment. Withdrawal of antiandrogen treatment often causes a paradoxical response.
- Chemotherapy is now used more. Docetaxel, given with prednisone, is the most effective regimen.
- Bisphosphonate treatment palliates bone metastases. Zoledronate by 3-weekly IV infusion is currently the most effective regimen.
- Radiotherapy is effective for bone pain and may pre-empt or reverse spinal cord compression.
- Treatment of local prostatic relapse can provide effective palliation.
- Radioisotope treatment with strontium-89 or other agents will relieve bone pain but not cord compression.
- Regular non-steroidal anti-inflammatory drugs (NSAIDs) should be the initial analgesic regimen for bone pain.

What is done when the PSA starts to rise is very much a matter for specialist decision. There is much controversy as to managing men in this situation; as already mentioned, it is tempting to treat the PSA rather than the patient. What intervention is appropriate will depend on the circumstances. For example, if the pathology of a radical prostatectomy specimen suggested a high chance of there being residual disease, radiotherapy to the tumour bed might be appropriate, whereas if systemic metastases were suspected, hormone treatment might be preferred. With a late, and slowly rising PSA, surveillance might still be appropriate in the absence of other evidence of recurrent disease.

Hormone refractory disease

Whether used as part of the initial management, or commenced after failure of other treatments, hormone treatment is the ultimate treatment for uncontrolled disease. Although effective in the short term, in time, hormone refractory disease will occur (see p. 95, 'Hormone treatment'). Its management is one of the disease's greatest challenges, and is the area on which most research into new treatments currently is focused. Biochemical (PSA) relapse usually precedes clinical evidence of disease progression by several months. It may be difficult to know how best to manage the patient, who will probably be symptom free, at this stage.

In addition to any change in therapy that might reverse or slow progression of the disease, it is important that any problems for which specific palliative treatment is needed are identified. The window of warning provided by the PSA rise gives an opportunity to reassess the patient and to determine whether, for example, relapse is due to local recurrence or to progression of metastatic disease. If the former, in a man who has not already received it, radiotherapy to the prostate may well prevent or delay the onset or deterioration of lower urinary symptoms or, more seriously, retention or ureteric obstruction. Similarly, identifying and treating a large destructive spinal metastasis might pre-empt cord compression.

Second-line hormone treatments

As the treatments described on p. 95 ('Hormone treatment') leave a small hormone drive to the prostate, there is always the possibility of a response to further reduction in hormone drive. This will usually mean prescribing the antiandrogen bicalutamide for the man receiving a luteinizing hormone releasing hormone (LHRH) analogue (or one who has had an orchiectomy); if bicalutamide has been first-line treatment, then an LHRH analogue could be started. Generally speaking, an additional hormone treatment is likely to be effective only if there has been a good response to the first-line treatment.

120

Antiandrogen withdrawal

If relapse occurs when a patient is on an antiandrogen, stopping the drug is often followed by a response, at least to the extent of a reduction in PSA level. This seems to be due to antiandrogens paradoxically having a mild androgenic stimulatory effect.

Chemotherapy

For many years, cytotoxic chemotherapy had little benefit in advanced prostate cancer. This was in part due to a lack of sensitivity to the agents then available. Also, in the days when relapse was diagnosed clinically at a late stage, patients were often not fit enough to cope with the toxicity of chemotherapy, particularly when they were elderly. Relapse can now be diagnosed at an earlier stage, and the disease is occurring in a fitter and perhaps younger population. Newer chemotherapy agents have been shown to be effective in prostate cancer. Mitoxantrone, in combination with prednisone, was first shown to be effective, not in prolonging life but in improving its quality. More recently, docetaxel in clinical trials has demonstrated an increase in actual survival. As a result men with hormone refractory disease are being increasingly offered chemotherapy treatment.

Bisphosphonates

As prostate cancer metastasizes to the skeleton predominantly, drugs which affect calcium turnover are effective in reducing the symptoms of, and complications from, metastases (*skeletal-related events*). Although older oral drugs are effective, zoledronate given by an IV infusion every 3 weeks, is the most powerful of the current agents.

Radiotherapy

Although radiation treatment has a key role in the management of late prostate cancer, it is essentially a palliative measure. It is the main method of controlling symptoms from bony metastases, although its use in controlling local relapse in the prostate, perhaps used insufficiently, is also important. Painful bone metastases will usually respond to local radiotherapy treatment, traditionally given in ten fractions, although a single treatment is effective and used now more frequently. Where pain is widespread, *wide field radiotherapy*, as it were bathing half the patient with a relatively low radiation dose (the bone marrow in the untreated half maintaining the blood count), can be used. To an extent this technique has been superseded by radioisotope treatment.

Promptly administered radiotherapy can pre-empt paralysis from impending spinal cord compression – indeed, if a bone scan identifies a hot spot, especially if there is radiological bone destruction, preventative radiotherapy may be appropriate, even if the lesion is asymptomatic.

Radioisotopes

The β-emitting isotope of strontium (Sr-89), which the body handles like calcium, is concentrated in the sclerotic metastases typical of prostate cancer. Equally effective to external beam treatment in relieving existing pain, the isotope is taken up by all the metastases, and there is evidence that this prevents or delays the onset of new sites of pain. Radioactive isotopes of rhenium and samarium are also used to treat metastatic prostate cancer. Radioisotopes have no protective effect against cord compression or pathological fractures and the patient must be carefully assessed by a radiation oncologist before treatment.

Palliative care

As with all cases of terminal cancer, effective palliative care is essential to maintain the quality of the last months of the patient's life. Since prostate cancer patients with symptomatic bone metastases can otherwise be quite fit, this stage of the disease can last for many months, during which pain relief is the main issue. A detailed account of palliative care is perhaps outside the scope of this book (or indeed the expertise of the author), but possibly elderly men dying from prostate cancer may have been neglected in the past in favour of younger people suffering from other forms of terminal cancer.

Choice of analgesics

However, both in primary care and in the urology and oncology departments, it is important to emphasize the effectiveness of non-steroidal anti-inflammatory drugs (NSAIDs) in managing pain from bony metastases. Frequently, symptoms for which radiotherapy is being considered can be brought under control by properly prescribed – i.e. regular doses of – NSAIDs, and even in more severe pain, regimens should be used based on NSAIDs with additional drugs for breakthrough pain.

19 ACUTE PROSTATITIS AND URINARY INFECTION IN THE MALE; PELVIC PAIN SYNDROMES

Management points

- Acute prostatitis may be confused with a simple urinary infection.
- Inadequate treatment may resolve symptoms, but leave residual infection which may flare up – a cause of 'recurrent urinary infections'.
- Treatment should be with a quinolone antibiotic for 4–6 weeks.
- 'Chronic prostatitis' is now called 'pelvic pain syndrome'.
- Pelvic pain syndrome is classified into infective and non-infective inflammatory and non-inflammatory causes.
- Distinguishing these can be difficult: therapeutic trials of quinolone antibiotics, anti-inflammatory drugs and α-blockers may be necessary.
- Asymptomatic inflammatory 'prostatitis' may be a source of recurrent urinary infections, and can also cause a spuriously high PSA.

Acute prostatitis

Acute infection of the prostate can occur at any age. Typically, there are severe urinary symptoms, frequency and dysuria, of sudden onset, with high fever and rigors. Less severe attacks may be mainly characterized by lower urinary symptoms, and be diagnosed as a 'UTI'. Typically, the prostate will be tender, and possibly feel 'boggy' on palpation. There will probably be pyuria, and there may or may not be growth on culture. In the older man with pre-existing outflow obstruction, it might precipitate retention of urine.

Adequate treatment is essential if relapsing disease is to be avoided, and indeed proper treatment may prevent the development of the type of problem discussed later in this chapter (see below 'Pelvic pain syndromes'). It has to be understood that in the prostate, antibiotic treatment is problematic for two reasons: poor penetration of the prostate by many antibiotics, and the low pH of prostatic fluid, when many antibiotics are only active in a neutral or alkaline environment. Treatment appropriate for 'cystitis' in the female may be inadequate for a urinary infection in a man.

The ideal antibiotic is one of the newer quinolones, ciprofloxacin, norfloxacin or ofloxacin. These should be administered in full dose, for at least 4 weeks. If for any reason treatment with one of these agents is not possible, trimethoprim can be used. While symptoms may well resolve rapidly, too short a course of treatment will not eradicate infection, and it may flare up in future: the usual cause of 'recurrent urinary infections' in men. Indeed, when a man does get repeated infections, even if not of full-blown prostatitis, treatment for 4–6 weeks with a quinolone may resolve the problem. In severe cases, emergency hospital admission for IV fluids, etc., may be needed.

A word of warning: this is not the time to measure PSA. Severe prostatitis can cause a marked elevation of PSA, which may persist for weeks, or even months. If there is concern about coincidental prostate cancer, the PSA measurement should be delayed until well after the event, and even then, if elevated, should be repeated to make sure it is not still falling.

A small proportion of men who develop a urinary infection or prostatitis will have a treatable underlying problem, and most men will find their way into the hands of a urologist. Referral is probably wise, although in the author's experience investigation of young men after a single urinary infection is usually unproductive. An ultrasound scan of the urinary tract is probably sufficient, reserving more invasive investigations such as cystoscopy for those whose symptoms recur despite adequate antibiotic treatment.

Pelvic pain syndromes

While chronic infection or abacterial inflammation of the prostate are real entities, indistinguishable symptoms occur without evidence of inflammation, and indeed may not necessarily arise from the prostate. Hence the term *chronic prostatitis*, which implies a specific aetiology, has been abandoned in favour of '*pelvic pain syndrome*'. The following classification, proposed jointly by the National Institutes of Health (NIH) of Canada and the USA, is now widely used.

- Type I is essentially acute prostatitis as described in the previous section.
- Type II is chronic bacterial infection of the prostate.
- Type III is pelvic pain without evidence of prostatic infection.
  Type IIIa is characterized by inflammation without demonstable bacterial infection.
  Type IIIb is non-infective and non-inflammatory – a condition previously described as 'prostatodynia'.
- Type IV is asymptomatic inflammatory prostatitis.
  This is often due to an occult infection. It has two important clinical consequences: a source of recurrent urinary infections and an increase in serum PSA. In either situation, the patient may benefit from a 4-week course of a quinolone antibiotic.

Typical symptoms are lower abdominal and perineal pain. Testicular pain and back and leg pain may also be features. Urinary symptoms as such are variable, and sometimes flare up intermittently on a background of chronic pain. Some men will complain of slow urinary stream. The patient is frequently anxious and introspective. It is often difficult to decide whether this is a consequence of the syndrome or antedates it, but certainly in some men stress can bring on or exacerbate the symptoms.

Management of these patients is one of the biggest problems most urologists encounter. Investigations are usually unhelpful, but do reassure the patient that he has no serious underlying disease (as always, there is often fear of cancer). To diagnose whether there is inflammation and infection requires examination of prostatic fluid. This can be obtained by prostatic massage, either collecting the fluid itself, or using the patient's urine to flush it out for comparison with a pre-massage urine specimen. This is very much something for the specialist, and not even done by many urologists. In most cases, therapeutic trial replaces rational investigation. This will start with a thorough attempt to eradicate any infection with quinolone antibiotics. Anti-inflammatories will help in some cases of type IIIa. Non-inflammatory (type IIIb) often benefits from α-adrenergic blockers (alfuzosin, tamsulosin, etc.). The rationale is that 'prostatodynia' results from spasm of the prostatic smooth muscle.

Sadly, these treatments are all too often found wanting. As with most intractable conditions, a variety of measures may be tried, among them massage of the prostate under general anaesthetic and steroid injections. Most important is general and sympathetic support of the patient. In intractable, severe symptoms, referral to a specialist pain clinic may be helpful.

These syndromes are now recognized as a neglected area of urology, and probably commoner than previously recognized. This neglect is at last being addressed by serious research. For example, is type IIIa (abacterial 'prostatitis') genuinely sterile or have we yet to identify an organism causing it? 'Watch this space' is the author's conclusion.

20   PROSTATE DISEASE: THE FUTURE

In the 1970s the author worked in an academic surgical unit, which was heavily involved in a clinical trial comparing various surgical operations for peptic ulcer disease. At the same time, a few patients were involved in testing a new drug for the same condition – about which there was some considerable scepticism. That drug was, of course, cimetidine and was the first step in a chain of developments that has more or less abolished surgical treatment of peptic ulcer disease. Similar scepticism has greeted medical treatment for benign prostatic hyperplasia (BPH), but it is likely that with increased understanding of its causes, this condition in its turn will leave the operating theatre.

What of prostate cancer? Can we improve our use of current treatments, develop new treatments and perhaps in the future even be able to prevent it?

As described on p. 94, 'Deferred treatment in early disease', distinguishing aggressive from indolent tumours (separating the 'tigers' from the 'pussy cats'), would avoid invasive treatment for those not at risk. The problem of hormone refractory disease has also been described. Resolution of both these issues will have to come from the laboratory, as will the development of drugs providing the benefits of hormone treatment without the current toxicity. Clinical research is needed to compare the merits of the various treatment options – despite its use for a century, we still can't with confidence advise our patients on the merits of radical prostatectomy, nor of its efficacy compared with alternative treatments. In a disease with such uncertainties, encouraging patients to participate in clinical trials is important.

Treatments for prostate cancer traditionally are used sequentially. Despite the disappointing performance of combined androgen blockade (see p. 99, 'Combined androgen blockade'), and the lack of clear survival data as yet for adjuvant bicalutamide treatment (see p. 108, 'Adjuvant hormone treatment'), benefits do seem to accrue from adjuvant hormone therapy after radiotherapy. Would the treatments currently in use for relapsed disease (chemotherapy, etc.) have benefits if used early? STAMPEDE is a large multicentre study in which a variety of treatments, presently used late in the disease, are introduced in combination when hormonal treatment is commenced.

There is a considerable amount of research into new treatments, from which, it must be admitted, little of practical use has yet to emerge. The prostate has some attractive features for innovation. It is readily accessible. Radical prostatectomy provides useful research material, and also enables the tissue effects of new treatments, administered in the pre-operative period, to be studied. Expression of unique genes related to production of PSA and other proteins should facilitate selective uptake of gene therapies. Other innovative treatments under trial include immunotherapy. For ethical and other reasons, new treatments are often introduced in the pre-terminal stage of a disease, when all other therapies have been exhausted. The comparatively long duration of this phase of the disease in prostate cancer allows time for assessment of new treatments.

Perhaps we can't improve treatment much. Screening to identify disease while it is still curable, as with breast and cervical cancer, is a topic of much debate. For reasons discussed in several sections of this book, the value of screening for prostate cancer remains uncertain. Would it really reduce the mortality? If so, would this be at the expense of over-treatment of many men whose disease, if undetected, would never have become clinically evident? The European Trial of Prostate Cancer Screening is designed to answer these questions – but at present how much population screening would reduce prostate cancer mortality is uncertain.

Can we prevent prostate cancer? Lifestyle can certainly influence its incidence. Its low incidence in Japan seems to be due to diet, probably the consumption of phyto-oestrogenic soya products. High-fat diets are associated with an increased incidence, and possible protective effects of tomatoes and other vegetables, vitamins and other dietary manipulations have been identified. Chemoprevention with a number of substances has been proposed. A large study using the 5α-reductase inhibitor finasteride demonstrated a reduction in the incidence of prostate cancer on biopsy in those on the drug. Whether this would translate into a reduction in the incidence of clinical disease and reduce mortality is less clear. There was also a higher proportion of high-grade tumours in those receiving finasteride, although this may be a histological artefact. It has not been suggested as a result of these data that finasteride should be prescribed for this purpose, nor should its use in managing BPH be modified.

Hereditary factors probably are important in many cases of prostate cancer. However, and despite much research into the genetics of the disease, as yet, specific prostate cancer susceptibility genes have proved elusive, and genetic testing for propensity to the disease is still a distant prospect.

Regarding current management, a notable change in urological practice in the past decade has been the increased role of nurses in areas previously the province of the surgeon. This applies both to BPH and to prostate cancer management, with nurses increasingly involved in care of patients, during diagnosis, counselling about treatment options, and in follow-up. Nurses are now beginning to perform prostate biopsies, a development which would become essential if prostate cancer screening was introduced.

Whatever the future holds, there is no doubt that the role of the primary care team can only increase. With increasing medical options for BPH, as with peptic ulcer disease, the hospital may simply become a supplier of diagnostic services. Prostate cancer will be an increasing issue, as the elderly population increases. I would predict that improved understanding of the natural history of the disease will increase the proportion of men under active surveillance, and where better for this than the man's local health centre? It may well even now be appropriate to consider enhanced contractual arrangements for managing prostate cancer in primary care, and as with other disease areas (e.g. dermatology, psychiatry) for there to be GPs with a special interest in prostate disease or indeed urology in general.

APPENDIX 1 PSA TESTING FOR PROSTATE CANCER*

The following is the text from an information sheet for men considering a PSA test.

What is the aim of this leaflet?

Prostate cancer is a serious condition. The PSA test, which can give an early indication that prostate cancer may be present, is now available to men who wish to be tested. However, experts disagree on the usefulness of the PSA test. It is not yet known whether or not PSA testing will save lives from prostate cancer. The aim of this information sheet is to give you balanced information about the PSA test, which we hope will help you decide whether or not having the test is the right thing for you.

You may wish to discuss this information with your doctor or practice nurse.

What do we know about prostate cancer?

Prostate cancer is the second most common cause of cancer deaths in men. Each year in the UK about 22 000 men are diagnosed with prostate cancer and 9500 die from the disease. Prostate cancer is rare in men below the age of 50 years, and the average age of diagnosis is 75 years. The risk is greater in those with a family history and is also known to be greater in African American men. Prostate cancer is also more common in the West, suggesting that there may be a link with western lifestyle factors, such as diet.

* The information sheet was prepared by Jo Brett, Dr Eila Watson, Colleen Bukach and Dr Joan Austoker, Cancer Research UK Primary Care Education Research Group, University of Oxford. The information sheet is based on information initially prepared by Dr Graham Easton. The information sheet is available from http://www.cancerscreening.nhs.uk/ prostate-patient-info-sheet.pdf.

The prostate gland lies below the bladder. Prostate cancers range from very fast-growing cancers to slow-growing cancers. Slow-growing cancers are common and may not cause any symptoms or shorten life.

- Prostate cancer is the second most common cause of cancer deaths in men.
- Prostate cancer is rare in men under the age of 50 years.

What is a PSA test?

The PSA test is a blood test that measures the level of PSA in your blood. PSA (prostate specific antigen) is a substance made by the prostate gland, which naturally leaks out into the bloodstream. A raised PSA can be an early indication of prostate cancer. However, other conditions which are not cancer (e.g. enlargement of the prostate, prostatitis, urinary infection) can also cause a rise in PSA.

Approximately 2 out of 3 men with a raised PSA level will not have prostate cancer. The higher the level of PSA the more likely it is to be cancer.

The PSA test can also miss prostate cancer.

- A PSA test involves a blood test.
- If the level of PSA in the blood is raised, this may indicate that prostate cancer is present.
- However, many men with a raised PSA will not have prostate cancer.
- The PSA test can also miss prostate cancer.

What happens after the PSA test?

As a rough guide there are three main options after a PSA test:

PSA level is not raised
- Unlikely to have cancer.
- No further action.

PSA slightly raised

- Probably not cancer, but you might need further tests.

PSA definitely raised
- Your GP will refer you to see a specialist for further tests to find out if prostate cancer is the cause.

If the PSA level is raised, what further tests would be carried out?

If your PSA is definitely raised, a prostate biopsy is required to determine if cancer is present. This involves taking samples from the prostate through the back passage (bottom). Most men find this an uncomfortable experience, and some describe it as painful. Sometimes complications or infection may occur. Approximately 2 out of 3 men who have a prostate biopsy will not have prostate cancer. However, biopsies can miss some cancers and worry about prostate cancer may remain even after a clear result.

- While a raised PSA level in the blood may indicate cancer, a prostate biopsy is still required to determine if cancer is present.
- About 2 out of 3 of men who have a biopsy will not have prostate cancer.

If early prostate cancer is detected, what treatments are used?

There are three main options for treating early prostate cancer which are summarized below:

- **Radiotherapy**: This involves a course of radiotherapy treatment on the prostate gland at an outpatient clinic. The aim is to cure, although there are possible side effects. Impotence (erection problems) may be suffered by between 2 and 6 out of every 10 men (25–60%). Up to 1 in every 10 men (10%) may experience diarrhoea or bowel problems, and up to 1 in every 20 men (5%) may experience bladder problems.

- **Surgery**: This involves an operation to remove the prostate gland. The aim is to cure, although again there are possible side effects. Up to 2 in every 10 men (20%) may experience some bladder problems, and between 2 and 8 out of every 10 men (20–80%) may experience impotence (erection problems) after surgery.
- **Active monitoring**: This involves regular check-ups to monitor the cancer and check it is not growing. The advantage is that for many men it avoids the side effects of radiotherapy and surgery. If there are signs that the cancer is developing, treatment would be offered. The disadvantage is that the cancer may grow to a more advanced stage. Some men find the uncertainty difficult to cope with.

So should I have the PSA test?

Benefits of PSA testing

- It may provide reassurance if the test result is normal.
- It may find cancer before symptoms develop.
- It may detect cancer at an early stage when treatments could be beneficial.
- If treatment is successful, the consequences of more advanced cancer are avoided.

Downside of PSA testing

- It can miss cancer, and provide false reassurance.
- It may lead to unnecessary anxiety and medical tests when no cancer is present.
- It might detect slow-growing cancer that may never cause any symptoms or shortened life span.
- The main treatments of prostate cancer have significant side effects, and there is no certainty that the treatment will be successful.

APPENDIX 2 TNM STAGING OF PROSTATE CANCER

TNM staging of prostate cancer

TNM	Description
Primary tumour clinical staging (T)	
Tx	Primary tumour unable to be assessed
T0	No evidence of primary tumour
T1	Tumour not apparent on palpation or imaging
T1a	Incidental finding at TURP (<5%)
T1b	Incidental finding at TURP (>5%)
T1c	Tumour identified at time of biopsy (PSA elevation)
T2	Tumour confined within the prostate
T2a	Tumour involves less than half a single lobe
T2b	Tumour involves more than one half of a single lobe
T2c	Tumour involves more than one lobe (bilateral)
T3	Tumour not confined to the prostate
T3a	Extension through the capsule
T3b	Extension into the seminal vesicle(s)
T4	Tumour fixed or invades adjacent structures excluding seminal vesicles (bladder neck, external sphincter, rectum, levator muscles, and pelvic wall)
Primary tumour pathologic staging (T)	
pT2	Organ confined
pT2a/b	Unilateral involvement
pT2c	Bilateral involvement
pT3	Extraprostatic extension
pT3a	Capsular invasion
pT3b	Seminal vesicle invasion
pT4	Invasion of contiguous structures
Regional lymph nodes (N)	
Nx	Regional lymph nodes not assessed
N0	No involvement of regional nodes
N1	Regional lymph node involvement

TNM	Description
Distant metastasis (M)	
Mx	Distant metastasis not assessed
M0	No distant metastasis
M1	Distant metastasis
M1a	Nonregional lymph node involvement
M1b	Bone involvement
M1c	Involvement of other distant sites

APPENDIX 3   A NOTE ON EVIDENCE LEVELS

In this age of evidence-based medicine, the reader may be interested in the supporting evidence for the text of this book. As will have been apparent, one of the difficulties in managing prostate disease, especially cancer, is the absence of high-quality data on which to base decisions.

There is level one evidence from clinical trials for the efficacy of licensed medical treatments for BPH. A randomized comparison of TURP vs watchful waiting for BPH was carried out in the USA, but the entry criteria questions its applicability to the majority of men who undergo the operation in the UK.

While the randomized Scandinavian Radical Prostatectomy study (see p. 105, 'Treatment options') demonstrated a survival benefit from surgery, the patients were recruited prior to the introduction of PSA tests, so the results may not be applicable to patients whose disease is now diagnosed at an earlier stage. The timing of hormone therapy has been controversial for over half a century, with clinical trials giving conflicting results although an unpublished meta-analysis does suggest that early treatment prolongs survival. The question remains as to whether the adverse effects of hormone treatment outweigh this benefit. There have been many trials comparing different hormone therapies. While it is accepted on the basis of randomized trial data that LHRH analogues are equivalent to orchiectomy and oestrogen treatment, the numbers in the trials really were too low to rule out the possibility of small but possibly significant differences. Patients with advanced disease were often too ill or had too short a life expectation to enter clinical trials, but with PSA to predict relapse after hormone therapy, it has now been possible to run good quality clinical trials of chemotherapy in advanced disease.

Those managing prostate cancer are only too aware of the deficiencies in the evidence base, and, perhaps late in the day, are working hard to rectify this. Screening for prostate cancer is the subject of a very large international European study. The UK ProtecT study is comparing prostatectomy, radiotherapy and active surveillance in screen-detected early prostate cancer, and a number of studies of different radiotherapy regimens, and of adjuvant hormone treatment are under way. However, the long time course over which early prostate cancer progresses means it will be many years until the results of these trials will find their way into clinical practice. Inevitably, current management is often based on 'expert opinion' (or, sadly, individual clinician's preferences or prejudices). In writing this book the author has tried to reflect the current consensus – if, however, his own prejudices have crept in, he can only apologize.

REFERENCES AND FURTHER READING

Further reading

Aus G, Abbou CC, Bolla M, Heidenreich A, Schmid HP, van Poppel H, Wolff J, Zattoni F. (2005) EAU guidelines on prostate cancer. *European Urology* **48**, 546–551.

British Association of Urological Surgeons guidelines for the management of metastatic prostate cancer (available on CD Rom from The British Association of Urological Surgeons, 35/43 Lincoln's Inn Fields, London WC2).

Kirk D. (2000) Open-access services in urology: the way forward. *Trends in Urology, Gynaecology and Sexual Health* **5**, 13–14.

Kirk D. (2002) Talking about benign prostatic hyperplasia. *Prescriber* **19 November**, 87–92.

LUTS suggestive of BPH. Series of articles published in *Trends in Urology, Gynaecology and Sexual Health*, 2005, **10**.

Madersbacher S, Alivizatos G, Nordling J, Rioja Sanz C, Emberton M, de la Rozette JJMCH. (2004) EAU (European Association of Urology) guidelines on BPH. *European Urology* **46**, 447–554.

Nickel JC. (2000) Prostatitis: lessons from the 20th century. *British Journal of Urology International (European Update Series)* **85**, 179–185.

Schröder FH, Gosselaar C, Roemeling S, Postma R, Roobol MJ, Bangma CH. (2006) PSA and the detection of prostate cancer after 2005. Part 1. *EAU-EBU Update Series* (supplement to *European Urology*) **4**, 2–12.

Speakman MJ, Kirby RS, Joyce A, Abrams P, Pocock R. (2004) Guideline for the management of male lower urinary tract symptoms. *British Journal of Urology International* **93**, 985–990 (also available on CD Rom from The British Association of Urological Surgeons, 35/43 Lincoln's Inn Fields, London WC2).

Summerton N. (2005) Prostate cancer follow-up in primary care. *Trends in Urology, Gynaecology and Sexual Health* **10**, 7–8.

Walker B, Kirby M, Kirk D. (2000) A private medical reveals a raised PSA. *Practitioner* **244**, 495–500.

Watson E, Jenkins L, Buckach C, Brett J, Austoker J. (2002) The PSA test and prostate cancer: an information pack for primary care (Prostate Cancer Risk Management Programme). Sheffield: NHS Cancer Screening Programmes.

Information books for patients

Kirk D. (2007) *Understanding prostate disorders.* London: Family Doctor Publications Ltd in association with the British Medical Association.

Cancerbackup. (2005) *Understanding cancer of the prostate.* Under revision – to be re-issued in 2007 as three separate booklets, each dealing with a different stage of the disease.

Mason M, Moffat L. (2003) *Prostate cancer: the facts,* Oxford: Oxford University Press.

Comprehensive textbooks

Kirby RS, Partin AW, Feneley M, Parsons JK (eds) (2006) *Prostate cancer: principles and practice.* London/New York: Taylor & Francis.

Kirby R, McConnell J, Fitzpatrick J, Roehrborn C, Boyle P (eds) (2005) *Textbook of benign prostatic hyperplasia,* 2nd edition. London/New York: Taylor & Francis.

INDEX

Note: page numbers in *italics* refer to 'Management points' and in **bold** to figures and tables.